Behavioral Neurology

Behavioral Neurology

JONATHAN H. PINCUS, M.D.

Associate Professor of Neurology
Yale University School of Medicine

GARY J. TUCKER, M.D.

Associate Professor of Psychiatry
Dartmouth Medical School

New York
Oxford University Press   London   1974   Toronto

This book is dedicated to our teachers, Gilbert H. Glaser and Thomas P. Detre, whose interests have stimulated our own.

"It ought to be generally known that the source of our pleasure, merriment, laughter, and amusement, as of our grief, pain, anxiety, and tears, is none other than the brain. It is specially the organ which enables us to think, see, and hear, and to distinguish the ugly and the beautiful, the bad and the good, pleasant and unpleasant. Sometimes we judge according to the perceptions of expediency. It is the brain too which is the seat of madness and delirium, of the fears and frights which assail us, often by night, but sometimes even by day; it is there where lies the cause of insomnia and sleep-walking, of thoughts that will not come, forgotten duties, and eccentricities. All such things result from an unhealthy condition of the brain."

Hippocrates

INTRODUCTION

It is a truism that the mind does not exist apart from the brain, yet the practice of categorizing diseases as "neurological" and "psychiatric" suggests otherwise. According to convention, neurology deals with "organic disease," that is, disease of the brain, in which symptoms can be closely correlated with specific alterations of brain structure or a disordered state of physiological or biochemical function. Psychiatry is designated as the province of "functional disturbances," which are defined as thought and behavior disorders that cannot be correlated with alterations of brain structure or biological function. The primary cause of functional disorders is traditionally related to stressful environmental influences. Hence the term "functional" carries the implication of reversibility. This division, however practical with reference to the proper referral of patients, obscures important aspects of behavioral disorders. It is incorrect to conceive of any disturbance of behavior or thought as "functional" because thoughts, feelings, and memories are as much the result of brain activity as movement, sensation, and speech. In addition, "functional" disturbances of intellect and behavior which result from environmental influences are often irreversible.

There is strong evidence that environmental influences at certain stages of life can produce permanent changes within the nervous system. One such change is amblyopia ex anopsia, a form of acquired blindness which affects infants and children who have uncorrected strabismus. Strabismus makes normal binocular vision impossible. To avoid double vision the child "suppresses" visual impulses arising from the weak eye by means of a cortical process which is not well understood. If the condition is not treated and the child is not forced to use the weak eye, permanent blindness in that eye develops. This form of blindness occurs commonly only in childhood, rarely if ever beginning in adulthood, despite the fact that adults with acquired weakness of extraocular muscles also frequently "suppress" the image which comes from the weak eye.

A similar condition has been reproduced in kittens. If the eyelid of the neonatal kitten is sewn shut for three months and then opened, vision is permanently lost in that eye. The same is not true for the adult cat. The cells of the visual cortex of the neonatal kitten are, like those of the adult cat, endowed with the ability to respond to patterns of light (angles or forms). Eyelid closure in the first three months of life results in the permanent loss of this cortical reaction, though normal retinal and geniculate responses to visual stimuli are retained. Thus, a cortical connection, present at birth, has been rendered permanently ineffective by environmental manipulation (Weisel and Hubel, 1965).

A possible analogy to this experiment may be seen in the work of Harlow and his associates (1971). Infant monkeys were taken away from their mothers and "raised" by surrogate mothers (rag dolls). Although they were healthy and well developed, showing no sign of abnormality in solving problems, these monkeys were unable to establish normal heterosexual relations even after transfer to a colony of normal monkeys. Partial and total social isolation during the first six months of life also led to severe, irreversible abnormalities in the adult monkey's behavior. The actual neurophysiological and neurochemical correlates of this state are not known. Isolation does not produce such abnormalities in older monkeys who have been raised by a normal mother.

These findings provide an experimental context in which the effects of early environment upon human development may be understood. Delay of motor and social development has been described in institutionalized infants who have been subjected to maternal deprivation in the first year of life. Though these children made dramatic gains when given the benefit of good maternal care starting in the second year, residual impairments which persisted at least through the preschool years were noted. Deficits were seen in their capacity for forming emotional relationships, in impulse control, and in areas of thinking and learning that reflect adaptive capacities and imagination (Provence, 1962). While the permanence of such deficits has not been fully demonstrated in humans, and genetic influences on the thought processes of previously institutionalized children have not been completely ruled out, it would appear that the human nervous system also has a potential for development that is largely determined by genetic factors but may be changed permanently by experience and is particularly susceptible to irreversible change during the first months and years of life.

Why is the immature nervous system so susceptible? In considering this question a brief account of the normal alterations in the brain that are known to occur early in postpartum life may be useful. The number of nerve cells does not substantially change after birth, yet brain size increases tremendously during the first year of life and does not fully complete its growth until adolescence. Two factors are primarily responsible for the enlargement of the brain during this period. One is the formation of myelin sheaths which facilitate axonal conducting and the other is the development of dendritic connections between nerve cells. The temporal association of myelin and dendritic development with the period of susceptibility of immature brain to environmental influences suggests that these factors may be related. If so, axonal conducting and myelin formation are likely to be less important than dendrite development in determining susceptibility to the environment. For axons have a more limited functional capacity and respond in an all or none fashion. Dendrites are capable of more prolonged and gradual electrical responses. Also there is evidence that functions of dendritic connections are developed in response to environmental influences during the period of rapid brain growth.

Axonal impulses are indistinguishable from animal to animal. Even the most sophisticated neurophysiologist would be hard pressed to tell if a propagated action potential came from the axon of a worm, a frog, or a human being. The major neurophysiological difference between species is not in the nature of nerve impulses but rather in the number of nerve cells and the type and number of dendritic connections between them. Similarly, the real difference between such sensations as pain, smell, and sight is not primarily determined by the pattern of axonal impulses.

The dendritic connections made by afferent nerves subserving the sensory organs, rather than axonal patterns, are what endow electrical messages with individual sensory significance. Intensity, however, is a function of the frequency of axonal impulses which in turn reflects the magnitude of the stimulus. Yet virtually nothing is known about the mechanism by which nerves make contact with each other. We do know that this is not a random process, but quite specific. Thus, a sensory nerve carrying information from a stretch receptor in the quadriceps muscle has synaptic contact with a motor nerve—not any motor nerve but the nerve which supplies that very same muscle. Though the factors involved in the organization of these connections are not known, they are clearly under genetic control. Considering that dendrites are a major determinant of the number and kind of contacts between nerve cells and consequently in the passage of neural information (impulses) from one cell to another surprisingly little is known about alterations of these structures in disease states. By means of a variety of standard histological techniques it is possible to stain cell bodies, axons, myelin, and glia, but it has been difficult for the pathologist to discern alterations in dendrites by light or electron microscopy.

Many disorders of nervous system functions are so incapacitating that one would expect to find histopathologic changes; yet in such disorders as idiopathic epilepsy, mental retardation, infantile autism, learning disorders, schizophrenia, and affective psychosis, no consistent histopathologic changes have been described that would indicate the etiology. This failure has contributed to the development of the concept of "functional" or "idiopathic" disease. The absence of lesions demonstrable by standard histological techniques has too often led to the assumption that no abnormality exists. Yet, in "idiopathic" epilepsy, electroencephalographic spikes, mainly dendritic in origin, are the laboratory finding which most consistently reflects abnormality (Brazier, 1958); and in Golgi-stained preparations from animals with experimentally induced epilepsy, neurons in the region of the epileptic focus (induced by alumina gel) have shown a striking loss of dendritic spines and other changes in dendritic structure (Westrum et al., 1965). There is also some evidence that a diminution in the number of dendrites may be correlated with severe mental retardation even in the absence of other changes (Huttenlocher, 1970).

Dendrites are activated in several different ways. One is through the release by a presynaptic cell of transmitter chemicals that act at the postsynaptic receptor site and are then rapidly inactivated or removed. Another is by hormonal secretion into the extracellular fluid of substances that influence general neuronal excitability by altering cellular metabolism and the membrane environment for longer periods of time than transmitters. Several chemicals are likely to be transmitters in the central nervous system—acetylcholine, norepinephrine, dopamine, serotonin, and possibly certain amino acids as well, e.g., gamma aminobutyric acid and glycine. Particular transmitter substances do not always have either an excitatory or an inhibitory effect; rather it is the nature of the interaction of transmitter with postsynaptic (dendritic) membrane that determines its action. Each nerve cell in the human brain receives messages from many other cells—some inhibitory and some excitatory. Each cell must average the sum of these effects in making the "decision" to fire.

There is growing evidence that disturbances in the synthesis, release, storage, and inactivation of transmitter substances and changes in the dendritic receptor sites at which they work may lead to profound neurological and behavioral changes. Although there are many more questions than answers, recent progress in this area has suggested that certain amino acids, which probably act as transmitters, play an important role in movement disorders, sleep disturbances, and psychotic states.

These advances have extended the interest of psychiatrists and neurologists into overlapping areas. Interest in the biochemical basis of Parkinson's disease and chorea leads inevitably to an interest in the chemical basis of depression, mania, and thought disorders, and vice versa, because disturbances in the metabolism of the same catecholamines have been demonstrated or are suspected to exist in all these disorders. Similarly, the student of schizophrenia must understand and be able to differentiate the schizophrenialike psychosis of epilepsy, drug-induced psychosis, and the many neurological conditions which are often mistaken for schizophrenia. Too often monographs on these subjects are narrowly tailored to a preconceived notion of what will interest a neurologist or a psychiatrist, one interest excluding the other.

This book attempts to explore the traditional border zone between neurology and psychiatry. Seizure disorders are discussed with special emphasis on psychomotor seizures and the cognitive and behavioral disturbances with which they may be associated. The role of the limbic system in the production of psychosis and episodic violence is explored. The symptoms of dementia are discussed in terms of anatomic locus and etiologic considerations. The evidence that schizophrenia is an organic disorder of brain function is presented along with criteria by which it can be distinguished from diseases that can cause similar symptoms. Affective psychoses, movement disorders, and narcolepsy are described with emphasis on their treatment. On the basis of what is known about the mechanism of action of drugs which influence these conditions, a tentative hypothesis concerning their etiology is proposed. Elements in the medical history and examination that are important in differentiating these conditions are stressed. Also included is a discussion of commonly misdiagnosed conditions with hints as to how they may be differentiated. Hysteria, hyperventilation syndrome, and headache are treated in this way.

The book has developed from a course the authors have given to medical students at the Yale University School of Medicine, and from formal and informal sessions with residents in psychiatry and neurology. Selected references to important original papers and review articles are included.

REFERENCES

Brazier, M. A. B. The development of concepts relating to the electrical activity of the brain. J. Nerv. Ment. Dis. 126: 303, 1958.

Harlow, H. F., M. K. Harlow, and S. J. Suomi. From thought to therapy: Lessons from a primate laboratory. How investigation of the learning capability of rhesus monkeys has led to the study of their behavioral abnormalities and rehabilitation. Am. Scien. 59: 538, 1971.

Huttenlocher, P. R. Dendritic development and mental defect. Neurology 20: 381, 1970.

Provence, S. and R. Lipton. Infants in Institutions. International Universities Press, New York, 1962.

Weisel, T. V. and D. H. Hubel. Extent of recovery from the effects of visual deprivation in kittens. J. Neurophysiol. 28: 1060, 1965.

Westrum, C. E., L. E. White, and A. A. Ward, Jr. Morphology of the experimental epileptic focus. J. Neurosurg. 21: 1033, 1965.

CONTENTS

Behavioral Neurology

Chapter 1

SEIZURE DISORDERS

It is difficult to provide a simple, concise, and yet all-encompassing definition of epilepsy. Definitions which rely on clinical phenomena usually refer to loss of consciousness and to tonic and clonic movements. While these are components of grand mal seizures, in some forms of epilepsy both are absent. In focal motor seizures, for example, consciousness may not even be impaired. In other forms of epilepsy such as focal sensory, petit mal, or psychomotor seizures, abnormal movement does not necessarily occur. To avoid these difficulties in defining the clinical condition, some neurologists have anchored their definition in physiology, describing seizure states as "paroxysmal depolarization shifts" or the "repetitive discharge of a hyperexcitable aggregate of neurons." While such electrical changes always accompany seizures of any kind, they are not always reflected in the electroencephalogram (EEG) and sometimes they occur in the absence of clinically apparent seizures.

The diagnosis of epilepsy is not usually difficult despite the lack of a completely satisfactory definition of the condition. After the diagnosis has been made, however, it may not always be clear how much of a patient's behavior can be attributed to epilepsy. Even with a patient who is known to have seizures and/or whose EEG suggests an epileptic tendency, there may be disagreement among competent neurologists as to the relation of abnormal behavior to a seizure state. In such cases, a therapeutic trial of anticonvulsants may appear to resolve the medical problem, but the pragmatic definition of epilepsy as "that which responds to anticonvulsants" involves post hoc reasoning which is scientifically weak.

ETIOLOGICAL CONSIDERATIONS
Idiopathic vs. Symtomatic

Epilepsy traditionally has been divided into two broad etiological categories: symptomatic and idiopathic. The term symptomatic epilepsy is applied to seizure disorders with an identifiable cause, such as encephalitis, tumor, trauma, or known metabolic disease. In these conditions seizures are considered to be a symptom of another disease. The term "idiopathic" epilepsy literally means seizure disorders which arise spontaneously and exist in the absence of other diseases of the nervous system. This term is too broadly used when applied to all convulsive disorders in which no cause has yet been identified, irrespective of the age or family history of the patient. Used indiscriminately, "idiopathic epilepsy" becomes a subterfuge when a clinician lacks a clear-cut diagnosis. Used properly, the term probably should refer to "inherited" epilepsy. Idiopathic epilepsy, by this definition, usually begins in childhood or adolescence, and a positive family history is most helpful in making a reliable diagnosis. In older patients with negative family histories, epilepsy "of unknown cause" should be labeled as such, and the onus for incomplete diagnosis placed on the doorstep of the clinician, not the patient's genes.

It must be recognized that the concept of idiopathic epilepsy actually is artificial. The epilepsy is surely the result of a physiologic dysfunction, but the biochemical or neuroanatomical locus of the abnormality is not yet known. In this sense idiopathic epilepsy is "symptomatic," that is, symptomatic of an unknown abnormality. A high proportion of the relatives of patients with idiopathic epilepsy have abnormal EEG's, yet most of these persons never have clinical seizures. Some patients who have idiopathic epilepsy also show other symptoms of brain dysfunction and have a history of events known to be associated with brain damage. Acquired brain damage may promote expression of the genetic trait and to the extent that it does the resulting seizures are "symptomatic" of brain damage. It is also true that even in symptomatic epilepsy the mechanism by which identifiable lesions cause seizures is not well understood. Not every patient with a brain tumor, for example, has seizures. In all epileptic patients, whether they have idiopathic or symptomatic epilepsy, seizures are not constant, even though the lesion may be constantly present and the electroencephalogram consistently abnormal. It seems likely that other factors must prevent seizures from occurring all the time in such cases. The complexity of these factors is implied by the great variety of circumstances which can precipitate seizures in susceptible individuals (see Table 1-1).

Table 1-1
Factors Which May Precipitate
Seizures in Susceptible Individuals

Hyperventilation
Sleep (usually within the first 30 min. or shortly before awakening)
Sleep deprivation
Sensory stimuli
    Flashing lights
    Reading-Speaking, Coughing
    Laughing, Touch, Pain
    Sounds (music, bells, etc.)
Trauma
Hormonal changes
    Menses, Puberty, Adrenal steroids
    ACTH
Fever
Emotional stress
Drugs
    Phenothiazines, Analeptics
    Tricyclic mood elevators, Butyphenones
    Antihistamines, Alcohol
    Excessive anticonvulsants

While no single factor has been identified as the primary cause of convulsive disorders, some are well known to influence seizure threshold (Tower, 1960). These include the availability of prime energy substrates such as glucose and oxygen, the ability of the brain to utilize them, the metabolism of amino acids and acetylcholine, the activity of the sodium pump, and the distribution of cations within the nerve and at the cell membrane.

The patient's age at the onset of seizures gives an important clue to etiology. Seizures beginning before the age of six months usually reflect birth injury, congenital defect of the nervous system, metabolic errors, or infectious disease. Seizures beginning between the ages of two and twenty are usually "genetic" in etiology (i.e., idiopathic). When seizures have their initial onset after the age of thirty-five years, vascular disease or tumor is likely to be present. Seizures seldom begin between the ages of twenty and thirty-five. When they do, trauma, drug abuse (particularly involving alcohol), and infection are common causes. Idiopathic epilepsy does not usually begin between these ages, but it may. Sometimes patients forget about convulsive episodes that occurred 10 to 20 years before. Whenever possible, the history should be confirmed by interviewing the patient's parents or other individuals familiar with his early years. Despite this reservation, it is a good rule to assume that any seizures beginning after the age of twenty probably result from some identifiable, possibly progressive, condition which should be diligently investigated.

GENETICS

It has been a long-standing clinical observation that epilepsy is more common among close relatives of epileptics than in the general population, in which the incidence is probably close to one per cent. More recently it has become quite clear that the genetic element in epilepsy is not a simple one because the incidence of the disease in first-degree relatives of epileptics is much lower than would be expected in an autosomal dominant disorder (50 per cent) and the incidence in the siblings of epileptics is lower than would be predicted for an autosomal recessive condition (25 per cent). Nonetheless, a dominant mode of inheritance for epilepsy with incomplete penetrance was postulated in an early paper by Lennox, Gibbs, and Gibbs (1940) on the basis of the electroencephalographic traits of the relatives of epileptics. In a series of papers on centrencephalic (petit mal) epilepsy, Metrakos and Metrakos (1961) reported that the prevalence of convulsions among the near relatives of patients with petit mal epilepsy was high: 13 per cent of parents were affected and 13 per cent of siblings. In more distant relatives the prevalence was lower. This finding indicates a strong hereditary tendency in centrencephalic epilepsy but does not reveal the actual mode of inheritance. Further data from the same study on the electroencephalographic trait have conclusively demonstrated a dominant pattern of inheritance. Between the ages of 4½ and 16½ approximately 45 per cent of the siblings of epileptics demonstrated the typical 3 cycles per second (cps) spike and wave abnormality. After 16½ years there was a sharp decline in the incidence of this abnormality; and before the age of 2½ years only 6 per cent had it. Of forty siblings of epileptics between the ages of 4½ and 7½, twenty, or exactly 50 per cent, had the spike-and-wave abnormality (Metrakos and Metrakos, 1961). This is what would be predicted if the electroencephalographic abnormality were transmitted as an autosomal dominant trait. Thus, the 3 cps spike-and-wave abnormality is the expression of an autosomal dominant gene with the peculiar characteristic of a very low penetrance rate at birth which rises to nearly complete penetrance for ages 4½ to 7½ and declines to almost zero after the age of forty. The study by Metrakos and Metrakos also revealed that the electroencephalographic abnormality is not always associated with convulsions; only about 25 per cent of those with the EEG abnormality actually had clinical seizures.

Acquired brain damage may be another factor that determines which individual with the genetic trait actually becomes epileptic.

Reviewing prenatal and perinatal hospital records of epileptic children, Lilienfeld and Pasamanick (1954) found an increased incidence of complications of pregnancy, birth, and neonatal development compared with nonepileptic siblings. On the basis of this evidence, they suggested that brain damage often caused epilepsy even in those cases with an hereditary epileptic tendency.

Bray and Weiser (1964) studied focal and temporal lobe epilepsy associated with focal, temporal, or central electroencephalographic discharges. They found the same hereditary pattern that Metrakos and Metrakos demonstrated in petit mal epilepsy. Diffuse electroencephalographic abnormalities such as bilaterally synchronous spikes or combinations of spikes and slow wave discharges were found in almost half the close relatives of the index cases. Both groups found that the closer the relative, the higher the prevalence of seizures and abnormal EEG's. Bray and Weiser's index cases were homologous for type and location of the electroencephalographic abnormality but not for seizure type. Like Metrakos and Metrakos, Bray and Weiser demonstrated a dominant genetic trait which is age-related and has a low penetrance in early childhood that rises to approximately 50 per cent in middle childhood and then drops in adult life. On the basis of these studies, it seems likely that idiopathic epilepsy is transmitted by an autosomal dominant gene whose penetrance varies with the age of the individual and whose expressivity is determined in part by the presence of brain damage.

Twin studies have buttressed this view of the inheritance of epilepsy. Lennox (1951) found the concordance rate for seizures in the monozygotic twins of epileptics to be 85 per cent as compared with 27 per cent in dizygotic twins. Inouye (1960) found the rates to be 54 per cent and 7 per cent respectively. He also found a concordance rate for electroencephalographic abnormalities of 77 per cent in the monozygotic twins and 22 per cent in the dizygotic twins. Similar results were reported by Marshall and his associates (1962).

No study has shown a rate of concordance for seizures or electroencephalographic abnormalities in monozygotic twins greater than 85 per cent. The question of why the theoretically expected rate of 100 per cent for monozygotic twins has not been reached is of great interest. While the age of the nonindex twins at the time of study and the completeness of the criteria used to determine monozygocity may influence the concordance rate, the presence of acquired brain damage in one twin is the factor most likely to have caused nonconcordance in some monozygotic pairs. The presence of brain damage in one monozygotic twin might lower his seizure threshold enough to give expression to the inherited epileptic gene. There is an increased incidence of neurologic complications in the multiple-birth-children, and it is not unreasonable to expect that acquired brain damage would be expressed as epilepsy only in the damaged twin. Such an explanation would be consistent with the previously cited findings of Lilienfeld and Pasamanick.

CLINICAL CLASSIFICATION

GRAND MAL seizures are characterized by total loss of consciousness and stereotyped motor activity. Initially there is a tonic stage during which the body stiffens and breathing stops. This is followed by a clonic phase characterized by rhythmic shaking of the extremities and trunk. This sequence may last for a minute or two and sometimes repeats. After the convulsions stop there is a postictal depression of consciousness including drowsiness, confusion, headache, and somnolence which may last from a few minutes up to a day or two. About 50 per cent of patients experience some sort of aura which usually precedes the attack. An aura is an integral part of the seizure. In fact, an aura must be considered to be a seizure even when it is not followed by a grand mal attack. Usually it is an ill-defined sensation of not feeling well; sometimes it is essentially a psychomotor seizure. Patients with focal lesions in the cortex are apt to have an aura which can be related to the damaged

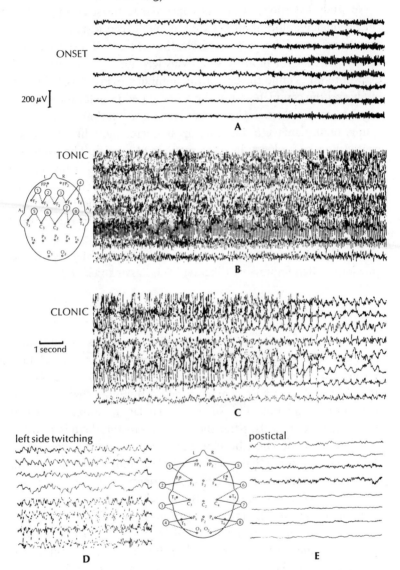

ONSET

200 μV

A

TONIC

B

CLONIC

1 second

C

left side twitching

postictal

D

E

area. Usually auras are of several seconds' duration but grand mal seizures may be preceded by prodromal periods of several hours' or even days' duration during which the patient does not feel well or is confused.

The tonic phase of a grand mal seizure coincides with generalized synchronous spikes on the EEG. The clonic stage is characterized by grouped spikes separated by slow waves. During the postictal phase low voltage slow waves are seen (*Fig. 1-1*). In about half the cases of grand mal seizures the interictal waking EEG is

FIG. 1-1

GRAND MAL SEIZURE WITH FOCAL FEATURES;
FOCAL SEIZURE AND POSTICTAL PHASE

A. The patient, a thirty-six-year-old man with post-traumatic epilepsy, had a generalized seizure during the recording. Irregular sharp waves from lines 1 and 5 are seen in the first EEG page (top). This abnormal activity derives from the left frontal and temporal regions. The background rhythms elsewhere are fairly normal. Generalized spiking then develops in all regions.

B. The second EEG page coincides with the tonic phase of the seizure. There is generalized, high-voltage spiking that is mixed with movement artifact from which it cannot be clearly distinguished.

C. The third EEG page coincides with the clonic phase of the convulsion and contains grouped spikes separated by slow waves. This feature of the record is best developed in lines 1, 2, 5, and 6, all of which are recorded from the left hemisphere. Clonic movements, though generalized, were more prominent in the right arm and leg.

D. These two EEG's are from another adult patient who had a right cerebral lesion. D was recorded during the clonic phase of a left focal seizure. Grouped spikes, separated by slow waves, can be seen in the right hemisphere. In the left hemisphere, slow waves predominate.

E. During the postictal phase E (the page on the right), there is a depression of amplitude and low-voltage slow waves in the leads from the right hemisphere which can be compared with the somewhat irregular but more normal activity in the left hemispheric leads. During this portion of the recording, the patient had a Todd's paralysis of his left arm and leg.

Ref Ipsi Ear

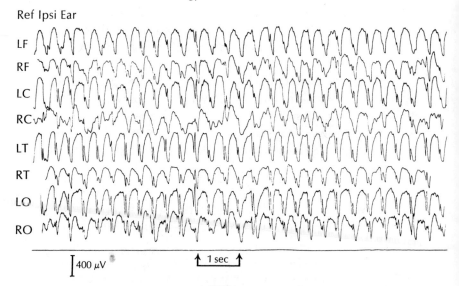

LF
RF
LC
RC
LT
RT
LO
RO

⌐400 μV   ↑ 1 sec ↑

FIG. 1-2

EEG record of a seven-year-old boy with a history of typical "absence" (petit mal) attacks usually lasting 5-20 seconds. The record shows generalized 3 cps spike-and-wave activity. In this illustration the spike-and-wave complexes are better developed in the left hemisphere.

LF left frontal, RF right frontal, LC left central, RC right central, LT left temporal, RT right temporal, LO left occipital, RO right occipital. Each electrode is referred to the ipsilateral ear.

normal. In the remainder, paroxysmal features including spikes, sharp activity, and slow wave bursts may be seen. If EEG's are recorded during sleep, abnormalities not seen in the waking EEG may be recorded but 25 to 30 per cent will still remain normal. Grand mal seizures may occur in the absence of any structural defect but may also be seen in patients with generalized or focal cerebral disease.

PETIT MAL (centrencephalic) seizures are characterized by "absence," a loss of awareness during which there is no motor activity other than blinking or rolling up of the eyes. The episodes are brief, usually lasting less than 10 seconds. Patients do not fall to the ground and there is no postictal depression. These seizures occur in children and are rarely seen in anyone over fifteen years old. Fifty to 75 per cent of patients with petit mal epilepsy do not have other types of seizures. The electroencephalographic pattern associated with petit mal seizures (in 80 per cent of cases) is the 3 cps spike-wave discharge (*Fig. 1-2*). The EEG is seldom normal in the interictal state, and it is especially sensitive to overbreathing. The term petit mal is often mistakenly applied to other forms of seizures, particularly psychomotor seizures, when some automatisms are present.

It has been thought that petit mal seizures result from a discharging focus in diencephalic structures. This might explain the bilaterally synchronous onset of the spike-and-wave discharge and close timing of the mirrored waves in homologous regions of the two cerebral hemispheres that occurs in petit mal, hence the term "centrencephalic." This view was substantiated to some extent by the finding that electrical stimulation of the thalamus in cats at 3 cps produces clinical and electroencephalographic phenomena similar to those of petit mal epilepsy (Hunter and Jasper, 1949). This classic experiment led to the hypothesis that an abnormal thalamic "pacemaker" exists in patients with petit mal. Similar clinical and electroencephalographic changes, however, have been produced in cats and monkeys by symmetrically placed epileptogenic foci in the cerebral cortex. In these experiments, a primary thalamic role in the production of epileptic phenomena was ruled out (Marcus and Watson, 1968). Thus, it remains unclear whether the thalamus is the major anatomical locus of abnormality in petit mal seizures. The condition may be the result of a genetically determined, diffusely altered state of excitability of cortical dendrites, synapses and/or cell bodies.

FOCAL seizures may be motor, sensory, or both. In patients over the age of ten years, they usually indicate focal disease in the side of the brain opposite the affected side of the body. Focal seizures may occur in the so-called "Jacksonian march," starting in distal parts of one extremity and moving proximally. The seizures are not necessarily associated with unconsciousness, but generally when they advance to both sides of the body, consciousness is lost (*Fig. 1-1D, 1-1E*). Very often in the postictal phase a phenomenon known as "Todd's paralysis" occurs. This is a transient paralysis of the affected part of the body which indicates that there probably is a structural abnormality in the opposite side of the cerebrum. Todd's paralysis may also follow grand mal seizures and it then might have the same focal significance. Certain metabolic abnormalities may give rise to focal seizures in the absence of any structural abnormality. Among these disturbances are hypoglycemia and hypocalcemia. Children in their first decade may have focal seizures in the absence of focal brain lesions.

MINOR MOTOR seizures are a category of epilepsy in which motor activity may be less dramatic and less prolonged than in other types but the disorder of the central nervous system associated with them is not necessarily minor. Minor motor seizures may be divided into three kinds:

INFANTILE SPASMS are massive myoclonic spasms that basically consist of a sudden flexion or extension of the body and often begin with a cry. These spasms may resemble an exaggerated Moro reflex. They usually begin between three and seven months of age and they are associated with an electroencephalographic pattern which is called hypsarhythmia. This term refers to a maximally abnormal EEG in which diffuse slow waves and spikes occur in a multifocal asynchronous pattern in all leads (*Fig. 1-3*). Nine of every ten children with infantile spasms become seriously retarded.

One of the striking aspects of this form of epilepsy is that conventional anticonvulsant therapy usually has no effect. ACTH came into use to control infantile spasms in the late 1950s and there were initial reports of success. The EEG was "normalized"

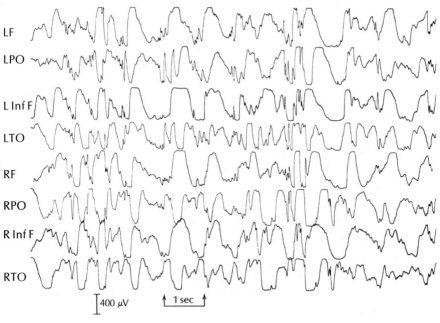

LF

LPO

L Inf F

LTO

RF

RPO

R Inf F

RTO

400 µV   1 sec

FIG. 1-3

EEG record of an 8½-month-old girl with infantile spasms. The diagnosis of tuberous sclerosis had been entertained on the basis of the family history. The record shows large slow waves and spikes which occur asynchronously and synchronously. Abnormal electrical activity is seen in all brain regions. LF left frontal, LPO left parieto occipital, L Inf F left inferior frontal, LTO left temporo occipital.

within days, the seizures stopped, and there was an apparent improvement in mentation. Subsequent follow-up studies indicated that, while ACTH often alleviates infantile spasms and "normalizes" the EEG, it has no effect upon ultimate retardation in the majority of cases, although by limiting the number of postictal depressions it does seem to brighten the patient intellectually. In isolated instances, early successful treatment has been correlated with satisfactory intellectual development, but the role of the hormone or the control of seizures in preserving intellect in such cases is not clear.

It is now known that many conditions can cause infantile spasms. Almost all of them have in common one characteristic: they cause a serious disruption of nervous system function. Diseases as diverse as phenylketonuria, hypoglycemia, subdural effusions, encephalitis, and congenital malformations of the nervous system all have been known to cause infantile spasms. These seizures, therefore, should be looked upon as the response of an immature nervous system to a serious insult. The retardation which accompanies this disorder is considered to be a result of the same insult. Generally, infantile spasms gradually resolve or else develop into some other clinical form. As the children grow older they often appear autistic. The reason ACTH is usually effective with infantile spasms irrespective of the disease causing them is not at all clear, for in older children and adults ACTH and adrenal steroids tend to be epileptogenic rather than the reverse (Bower and Jeavons, 1961).

In an AKINETIC seizure the child appears to fall to the floor passively without warning. His antigravity muscles seem to have relaxed. These spells may be of very short duration and after two or three seconds the child may get up quickly without any postictal depression. Akinetic seizures, however, are probably not actually akinetic, but rather myoclonic; they often result from active flexion of the neck and hips. The fall forward in the standing or sitting position may result in injury to the head and face (*Fig. 1-4*). Until such seizures can be controlled with medication these patients must sometimes wear football helmets to protect the face and head. Akinetic spells usually first occur in children between one and seven years of age. While these seizures may be seen in association with petit mal epilepsy, and as a manifestation of idiopathic epilepsy, most cases are associated with brain damage and have a poor

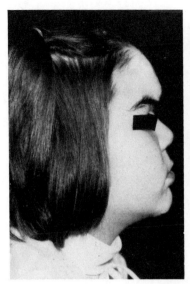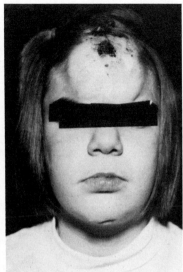

FIG. 1-4

An eight-year-old, educably retarded child with "akinetic" seizures which started at twenty months of age after an attack of encephalitis. Myoclonic flexion of her head and trunk over the years resulted in multiple facial injuries with scarring of chin, lips, nose, and forehead.

prognosis for normal intellectual development. They may thus be seen as a counterpart of infantile spasms in an older age group.

Akinetic seizures are often associated with an EEG pattern of spike-and-wave discharge which differs in frequency and form from the typical petit mal type. Hence, it is referred to as "atypical" spike wave (*Fig. 1-5*).

MYOCLONIC JERKS involving smaller muscle groups than the flexors and extensors of the hips may occur alone or as a prodrome to grand mal seizures. In either case they may also be a part of a mild idiopathic seizure disorder and are not necessarily an ominous sign. Myoclonic jerks occasionally occur in healthy individuals as they are falling asleep. This is called sleep myoclonus and it is a normal

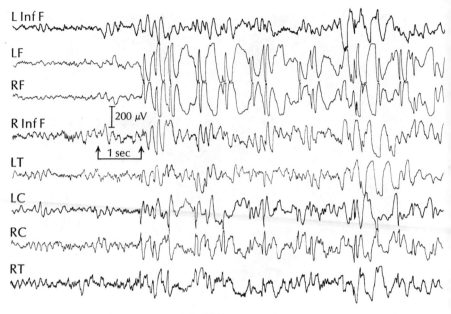

FIG. 1-5

EEG record of a mentally retarded 4½-year-old boy with grand mal seizures, psychomotor seizures, and akinetic spells. There is a strong family history of epilepsy. The record shows spikes, polyspikes, and atypical spike-wave combinations mainly in the frontal region which occur abruptly on a fairly normal background. Seizure activity begins under the EEG page number 185.

phenomenon. Myoclonic jerks are not always associated with non-progressive disorders, however. They occur in degenerative, infectious, and progressive diseases such as myoclonus epilepsy of Unverricht, subacute sclerosing panencephalitis (Dawson's encephalitis), storage diseases, and in certain metabolic disorders (i.e., uremia).

The terms PSYCHOMOTOR SEIZURES and TEMPORAL LOBE EPILEPSY are often used synonymously. Like many oversimplifications, this is largely correct: discharges that produce psychomotor seizures usually but do not always originate in deep, medially placed nuclei in the temporal lobe, which consists of the amygdala, uncus and hippocampus. They may also arise from virtually any other part of the limbic system, not all of which is located in the temporal lobe (q.v. ch. 2). In addition, other areas of the nervous system may be the source of the discharges causing psychomotor seizures. These discharges may arise from subcortical, frontal, diencephalic, or upper brain-stem regions and then spread through one or both

FIG. 1-6

EEG record of a forty-six-year-old man with psychomotor seizures. There are well-localized left anterior temporal spikes.
L Ant T left anterior temporal.

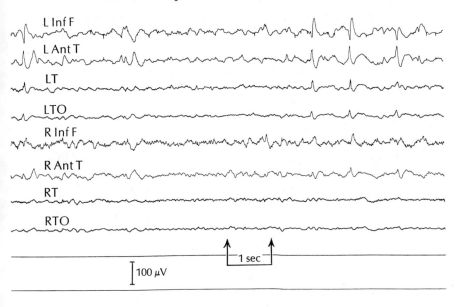

temporal lobes. In most cases, however, electrical activity spreads to the temporal lobes so that the characteristic electroencephalographic abnormality is temporal spiking (*Fig. 1-6*), unilaterally or bilaterally. Nonetheless, there are no pathognomic electroencephalographic configurations that make a diagnosis of psychomotor seizures absolutely certain, and the resting EEG may sometimes be normal.

The manifestations of psychomotor seizures fall usually into three categories: subjective experiences, automatisms, and postural changes. Autonomic changes also occur. The SUBJECTIVE FEELINGS include forced, repetitive, and disturbing thoughts, alterations of mood, sensations of impending disaster and anxiety, as well as inappropriate familiarity or unfamiliarity (*déjà vu, jamais vu*). Some patients have episodes of depersonalization, dreamlike states or sensations like those of alcoholic intoxication. Visual distortions such as macropsia and micropsia, auditory distortions, olfactory and gustatory hallucinations, and abdominal pain, are some of the most common sensory experiences. Abdominal pains associated with psychomotor seizures may be so severe as to simulate acute abdominal emergency and in some cases exploratory laparotomies have been performed.

The AUTOMATISMS of psychomotor seizures are much more difficult to recognize as ictal events than the tonic-clonic stages of a grand mal seizure. They tend to be repetitive and often are oral activities such as lip-smacking, chewing, gagging, retching, or swallowing. Some patients may perform a variety of complicated acts which seem to blend with normal behavior. Usually the behavior is inappropriate. The repetition of a phrase over and over again and the buttoning and unbuttoning of clothing are common. A few patients may assume bizarre postures resembling those of catatonic schizophrenia. These positions are held for variable periods of time. Some patients have fugue states. Fortunately, outbursts of directed, aggressive behavior are extremely rare, but when these outbursts lead to violence, they often present neurologists and psychiatrists with difficult medico-legal questions concerning the responsibility of an individual for his actions. Although the behavior of patients during psychomotor seizures tends to be automatic, it may be influenced by environmental factors. This influence can be seen in the case of a patient who had a psychomotor seizure while he was waiting in line at the hospital pharmacy to have his anticonvulsant prescription filled. It was a hot day and he was frustrated by the long wait. During the seizure he shoved past the people who were in front of him until he came to the pharmacist's window where he stood, mumbling incoherently until his wife led him away. After a minute or two of confusion, his sensorium cleared.

Sometimes it is quite difficult to distinguish behavior caused by psychomotor seizures from episodic aberrations caused by hysteria or even psychosis. In making this distinction six questions regarding the patient's history are especially helpful: (1) Does the patient describe subjective alterations typical of psychomotor seizures? (2) Has he been observed performing any of the characteristic automatisms? (3) Was he seen to be confused during the episode? (4) Is the patient's memory for events which occurred during the episode impaired? While memory for the early events of the seizure may seem relatively well preserved, such memories are nearly always incomplete or incorrect. (5) Did the patient experience a postictal depression? While such a depression is almost always present, it may be mild, and close questioning is often necessary to elicit a positive history. After the seizure, this depression may be manifest as only a brief period of fatigue, when the patient may wish to lie down, perhaps complaining of a headache or of not feeling quite normal. (6) Has he had other lapses during which he engaged in nearly identical behavior? Motor activity tends to be stereotyped in psychomotor epilepsy.

In some cases of psychomotor epilepsy there may be prolonged episodes of abnormal behavior lasting for hours or days. Although epilepsy is very rarely manifested solely as a prolonged behavioral disturbance, the clinician should include some form of associated seizure disorder in his differential diagnosis when considering episodic and especially patterned behavioral abnormalities even when they are prolonged.

In addition to the above criteria for establishing a diagnosis of psychomotor epilepsy, the EEG and the response to anticonvulsant therapy may aid in establishing a diagnosis. The EEG may help to confirm the suspicion that an active seizure state exists. It also provides information that helps determine whether a disorder is diffuse, lateralized, or focal in origin. The characteristic abnormality in psychomotor seizures is an anterior temporal spike focus, but in the waking state at least half the patients have a normal EEG (Gibbs and Gibbs, 1952). Repeating the test during sleep or using sphenoidal leads will reveal abnormalities in most patients, but still the incidence of normal records remains relatively high. Depending upon the criteria used for the diagnosis of epilepsy, normal sleep records may be seen in roughly one-third of epileptic patients. For this reason activating agents such as metrazol and megimide have been used to induce electroencephalographic changes in suspected epileptics. Though this is often successful, results must be interpreted cautiously as these drugs, even in low doses, may induce changes in some nonepileptic persons. If a normal EEG does not rule out psychomotor epilepsy, neither can the diagnosis of epilepsy be sustained merely on the basis of an abnormal record as 10 to 15 per cent of the general population have abnormal EEG's. However, these abnormalities usually are not of a paroxysmal or epileptiform type.

The use of a pharmacologic response to establish a clinical diagnosis is difficult at best and often impossible, yet a trial of anticonvulsant therapy starting with diphenylhydantoin may sometimes provide useful diagnostic information. In such therapeutic trials increasing doses should be given until either the seizures stop or signs of overdosage develop. Nystagmus is usually the first sign of toxicity with diphenylhydantoin, but not always. Other signs of toxicity include slurred speech, ataxia, lethargy, difficulty concentrating and dysmnesia.

PRINCIPLES OF THERAPY

The major principles of therapy for epilepsy are simple. Initially a single drug should be used at a moderate dosage. Then, the dosage should be increased until either seizures are controlled or toxic symptoms appear. If it is not possible to control seizures at nontoxic doses, a second drug should be added. A word of caution is called for here. If an epileptic patient begins to manifest behavior that is deemed undesirable by either the physician or the family, there is a tendency to interpret this behavior as part of the seizure problem and to increase the anticonvulsant medication. In an attempt to bring the behavior under control, drug dosages may be increased enough to produce a toxic state that worsens the behavior, and may lead to another increase in the medication and so on. Frequently, the only intervention that needs to be made at this point is to reduce the medication. The development and utilization of tests to determine the blood levels of the various medications, particularly diphenylhydantoin and phenobarbital, should mitigate this problem in the future. The determination of blood concentrations is of great help in determining whether or not a patient is taking his medicine as prescribed and whether more or less need be administered. Aside from the usual symptoms of toxicity with diphenylhydantoin (cerebellar symptoms, nystagmus, ataxia, sedation, euphoria) when the serum level of the drug is above 20 ug/ml, various psychiatric symptoms such as dementia, depression, and psychosis can develop. In some instances seizures even increase. Milder behavioral symptoms that are commonly described by patients with high diphenylhydantoin blood levels include feelings of lower energy levels and initiative, and decreased sociability and ability to concentrate.

Occasionally complete seizure control is not possible without some degree of toxicity. In such cases the functional capacity of the patient should determine what is an acceptable degree of seizure control. In general, amongst adult epileptics grand mal seizures are easiest to control and psychomotor seizures are the most difficult.

For a brief summary of the major indications for and uses of the usual antiepileptic drugs, see Table 1-2.

TABLE 1-2

Commonly Used Anticonvulsants

1. DIPHENYLHYDANTOIN (Dilantin, Phenytoin) is one of the most commonly used drugs particularly in adults for the control of grand mal, focal, and psychomotor seizures. It is essentially ineffective in petit mal and myoclonic seizures. Determination of the serum level of diphenylhydantoin in medical centers where the test is available provides a valuable guide to the adequacy of therapy; levels between 10 and 20 ug/ml are usually considered to be within the therapeutic range. There is considerable variation in the dosage necessary to achieve this—in some adults 200 mg is sufficient, others require 600 mg.

2. PHENOBARBITAL is the most commonly used of all seizure medications and is one of the most effective. It may be effective in all types of seizure disorders, including petit mal. The therapeutic serum level for phenobarbital is usually the same as for diphenylhydantoin though tolerance is demonstrated by some patients who have been receiving the drug for long periods of time, by which time they can tolerate much higher levels. Most hospitals are equipped to perform determinations of serum barbiturates in their routine laboratories.

3. PRIMIDONE (Mysoline) is a barbituratelike compound which has its greatest use in the control of psychomotor seizures. Though many neurologists feel it is more efficacious than phenobarbital in controlling psychomotor seizures, there is little published evidence indicating that this is so.

4. ETHOSUCCIMIDE (Zarontin) is the drug of choice in petit mal. It has little other use but may occasionally help out in minor motor seizures.

5. ACETAZOLAMIDE (Diamox) is a carbonic anhydrase inhibitor and may be effective in all seizure disorders, especially in minor motor

and petit mal seizures. High doses (30 mg/kg) are often necessary for seizure control.

6. DIAZEPAM (Valium) has been effective in some minor motor-seizure disorders when taken orally but is most useful when used intravenously in the treatment of status epilepticus. It has become the drug of choice to be used if intravenous barbiturates fail in treating status epilepticus.

7. TRIMETHADIONE (Tridione) is a fairly toxic compound useful for the same disorders as ethosuccimide.

8. QUINACRINE (Atabrine) is an antimalarial drug which is sometimes effective in petit mal and minor motor seizures. Although very safe, it turns the skin yellow and thus makes the patient look "different."

9. PARALDEHYDE, CHLORAL HYDRATE, AMYTAL, and the short acting barbiturates are sedatives useful only in status epilepticus.

10. STEROIDS AND ACTH are useful in infantile spasms and juvenile minor motor seizures at times. In other seizure types and at other ages these are epileptogenic.

11. THE KETOGENIC DIET is useful in difficult cases of minor motor seizures although it is somewhat complicated and unpalatable. It may completely stop seizures in 50 per cent of cases in which all other drugs have failed.

There are very few seizure disorders which will not respond to some combination of medications, but a small number of unfortunate individuals suffer from severe seizures that cannot be controlled by medical therapy. Surgical removal of focal epileptogenic tissue may help some of these patients, but cases need to be carefully selected. The primary criterion for surgery is the presence of a discrete focal lesion in an otherwise normal nervous system. Even afer surgery, many patients require anticonvulsant medication, albeit at lower dosage. When surgery is performed on epileptics with diffuse involvement of the nervous system it usually fails to control the seizures.

PERSONALITY, INTELLECTUAL DETERIORATION,
AND PSYCHOSIS IN EPILEPSY

It is well known that different parts of the hippocampus, particularly Ammon's horn are especially susceptible to reduction of energy production by such conditions as asphyxia, carbon monoxide poisoning, respiratory failure, and hypoglycemia (Green, 1964). Possibly as a consequence of this susceptibility, the hippocampus has the lowest seizure threshold of all cortical regions. A loss of neurons in this region is commonly seen in the brains of epileptics and it is thought that such changes result at least in part from the anoxia associated with seizures (Margerison and Corsellis, 1966). However, these lesions in the hippocampus may also give rise to seizures, particularly psychomotor seizures, as well as a variety of behavioral disturbances (Ounsted et al., 1966). The fact that there are lesions in these cases makes it reasonable to suppose that some form of deterioration of intellect and personality might occur in epilepsy and that such changes would be more often associated with psychomotor epilepsy.

Traditionally many personality characteristics have been attributed to epileptics. They have been described as paranoid, preoccupied with religion, prone to aggressive outbursts, pedantic, egocentric, perseverating (sticky), and obsessive. Very few patients combine all of these traits, which clearly are also present in other conditions. Consequently, these personality characteristics are of little clinical use.

To measure intellectual deterioration in epileptics, it would be necessary to control many factors such as the age of the patient at onset of seizures the duration of epilepsy, the clinical form of epilepsy (including the etiology and presence or absence of brain damage), the presence of other diseases, the social class and intelligence of the patient before disease onset, the drug used and its dosage and blood level, the frequency of seizures, and finally the length of time between the last seizure and the examination. It hardly needs to be said that the perfect study has yet to be done.

On the Wechsler Adult Intelligence Scale (WAIS) most epileptic patients have scores in the normal range, but the scores do tend to cluster around the lower end of the range (Rodin, 1968). This data is consistent with the theory that deterioration may occur in epilepsy but gives no information concerning the effect of repeated seizures and of different types of seizures upon the epileptic.

Obviously longitudinal studies are preferable in ascertaining intellectual deterioration, but very few of them have been done. Using the Wechsler Intelligence Scale for Children (WISC), Rodin (1968) studied the intellectual development of 58 epileptic children with follow-up testing after two years. He found that seizures were indeed related to a decrease in the I.Q., particularly on the performance scale. The deterioration was unrelated to the presumed etiology of seizures or to the presence of brain damage and it occurred mostly in patients who initially had above average I.Q.s. Rodin concluded that patients with complete seizure control did very well compared to those with incomplete seizure control but patients who had many seizures did not necessarily do poorly as compared with those who had fewer seizures. Although Rodin emphasized that deterioration was not necessarily permanent but rather reflected the state of affairs at the moment the patient was tested, his study showed quite clearly that incomplete control of seizures as such does correlate statistically with I.Q. deterioration.

Similar findings were recorded by Chaudhry and Pond (1961), who studied the role of major and minor seizures in intellectual and social deterioration. Twenty-eight epileptic children whose intellectual and social deterioration had been determined by serial testing and observation were compared with an equal number of epileptics who were matched for age, sex, type of epilepsy, and brain damage but who showed no deterioration. In the first group seizures were more frequent, the response to anticonvulsant medication was poorer, and abnormal electroencephalographic records were more common. No significant difference between the two groups was found in the ages at which brain damage had been sustained, the age of the patient at onset of epileptic attacks, the site or extent of brain damage, the amount or duration of anticonvulsant treatment, or family history of epilepsy. Like Rodin, Chaudhry and Pond emphasized that the deterioration in social and intellectual functioning was not always permanent; they also put forward the hypothesis that some "subclinical" form of seizure might be responsible for the apparent worsening in the clinical status of the patients who deteriorated. In this way the authors tried to explain the phenomenon of deterioration in patients who had relatively infrequent clinical seizures. While these studies are not conclusive they do support the impression that poorly controlled seizures cause temporary and sometimes permanent deterioration of intelligence.

Anoxia has been frequently suggested as the basic mechanism in epileptic deterioration. There is no doubt that tissue anoxia can occur in all forms of epilepsy and may be an important factor in deterioration. One would expect this to be an especially important factor in grand mal seizures, in which excessive muscular activity and apnea coincide with a generalized increase in neuronal firing rate which creates a metabolic demand that cannot be met. There is reason to believe, however, that anoxia is not the only causative factor in either chronic deterioration or postictal depression (a phenomenon which may be analogous and which is easier to study). There are as yet no firm indications of what the other factors may be—an embarrassing hiatus in medical knowledge. Todd's paralysis, for example, is a temporary paralysis that may occur after generalized seizures associated with prolonged anoxia but may also occur after brief focal seizures during which consciousness is preserved and respirations are normal. Impairment of recent memory following electroconvulsive therapy (ECT) in many nonepileptic patients occurs even when muscular activity during the ECT-induced seizure is abolished with succinylcholine and respiration and oxygenation are artificially maintained. After many shocks this transient deficit may become permanent in some cases.

If anoxia and subsequent metabolic changes such as buildup of CO_2, lactate, and a fall in pH were the only factors in determining postictal depression, and if epileptic deterioration were related to the same factors, patients with grand mal seizures would probably demonstrate greater intellectual deficits than those with psychomotor seizures. This prediction does not conform to the clinical facts (Guerrant et al., 1962). In addition, recent experiments have cast serious doubt on the accuracy of the theory that anoxia and other metabolic changes consequent to it are the only important factors in postictal neural dysfunction. Even when oxygenation was maintained and large accumulations of CO_2 and organic acids were prevented, electrically induced seizures still produced neuronal "exhaustion" in animals and humans during the postictal phase (Posner et al., 1969).

RELATIONSHIP OF SEIZURE DISORDERS
TO PSYCHOSIS

The role of seizures in the development of psychiatric disorders has been even more difficult to document than the intellectual deterioration they may cause, yet much has been written about the relationship between psychomotor seizures, or temporal lobe epilepsy, and psychosis. This may be explained by the widespread clinical impression that patients with psychomotor seizures are more prone to develop psychosis than patients with other forms of epilepsy.

In a study designed to test the hypothesis that patients with psychomotor seizures more often have psychiatric disorders than patients with grand mal epilepsy or non-neurological chronic illnesses, Guerrant and his colleagues (1962) studied 32 patients with psychomotor epilepsy, 26 patients with idiopathic grand mal epilepsy and 26 patients with a variety of chronic medical illnesses that did not involve the brain. The groups were fairly homogeneous in terms of age, sex, education, and social class, but the patients with psychomotor seizures received more anticonvulsant drugs than those with grand mal seizures and this factor was not adequately controlled. On independent evaluation by two psychiatrists, 47 per cent of the patients with psychomotor seizures were diagnosed as having an organic brain syndrome on the basis of impaired memory, attention, concentration, lability of affect, and slowed speech. Only 27 per cent of those with grand mal seizures and 4 per cent of those with a general medical illness were judged to have organic brain syndromes. Psychosis was also much more common in the group with psychomotor seizures. It was seen in 20 per cent of patients with psychomotor seizures and in only 4 per cent of those with grand mal. The incidence of psychosis in the general population is about 1 per cent (Srole et al., 1962). As the patients in Guerrant's study came from a low social class, the incidence rate of 20 per cent may be somewhat inaccurate for psychomotor seizures in general but the main point is clearly made.

Standard psychometric testing by Guerrant's group, however, failed to confirm the finding of increased abnormality in patients with psychomotor seizures. This discrepancy between the clinical impression of organic mental dysfunction and psychosis, on the one hand, and conventional psychological test results on the other has been the experience of several other investigators (Small et al., 1962). It may well be that the standard psychological tests used dealt with different aspects of cognitive and other psychological functions than the clinical interviews.

Although there had been many anecdotal reports linking schizophrenia and epilepsy (and occasionally even indicating their non-association), it was not until publication of a large study by Slater and Beard (1963) that a clear relationship between a psychosis resembling schizophrenia and epilepsy was established. Of 69 psychotic epileptics in this study, 80 per cent showed evidence of temporal lobe dysfunction on the basis of a history of psychomotor seizures and/or temporal lobe spiking on the EEG. The mean age of onset of psychosis was thirty years. The mean duration of the epilepsy before the onset of psychosis was fourteen years. Seizures varied from rare to frequent. However, all patients had incomplete seizure control at the time they became psychotic. There seemed to be no relationship between the onset of psychosis and the dosage of anticonvulsant drugs. It is highly unlikely that there could have been a chance correlation of epilepsy and schizophrenia in these cases. The ease with which the authors were able to collect 69 cases from the population served by their hospitals and the low incidence of schizophrenia in the first degree relatives of these patients are strong indications that they were suffering from something other than classic schizophrenia. While this group did show, at various times, all the cardinal features of schizophrenia, their psychoses deviated from norms for schizophrenia in some respects. Affective responsiveness was often preserved to an extent unusual in schizophrenia. In the later stages of the development of psychosis, the patient's personality was sometimes left essentially undamaged, which is rarely the case in the later stages of schizophrenia.

Slater and Beard, however, felt that the psychosis could not be symptomatically differentiated from ordinary schizophrenia without reference to historical material. In fact, two-thirds of the patients who had previously come into contact with independent psychiatrists were diagnosed as schizophrenics. Slater and Beard's study strongly suggests that epileptic psychosis can exist as a clinical entity which is etiologically distinct from schizophrenia. Furthermore, the study supports the contention that patterns of abnormal activity in the temporal lobe and its limbic projections predispose an individual to a schizophreniclike syndrome. This conclusion has been supported by other studies of psychotic epileptics (Pond, 1957; Glaser et al., 1963; Flor-Henry, 1969, 1972).

Other forms of mental abnormality have also been reported to coexist with epilepsy, and especially with psychomotor seizures. The association of psychomotor seizures with depression, hysteria, and aggressiveness has been less impressively documented, however, than the schizophrenialike psychosis of epilepsy. The evidence of such associations is essentially limited to case reports.

Some authors have commented on the tendency of some patients to become psychotic when seizures are controlled and vice versa (Pond, 1957; Flor-Henry, 1969; Reynolds, 1971). The only two studies which systematically directed attention to this observation are in disagreement.

Comparing 50 temporal lobe epileptics with psychosis to 50 without psychosis, Flor-Henry (1969) found that the number of psychomotor seizures was inversely related to psychosis. His psychotic patients had fewer psychomotor seizures or none at all, yet the incidence of major convulsions and the type of medication and dosage was similar in each group. Neurologic signs and abnormal EEG's (lateralized to the dominant hemisphere) were more prominent in the psychotic group, thus suggesting qualitative differences between the groups which were not controlled. In Slater and Beard's study, there was no relationship between severity or frequency of seizures and the development of psychosis in the great majority of the patients. In six cases psychotic symptoms appeared when the seizure frequency was falling and in two there was an increase in the seizure frequency shortly before the appearance of psychosis.

The etiology of the schizophrenialike psychosis of epilepsy is not known, but in considering the various possibilities in most patients with epileptic psychosis two clinical findings stand out: (1) a history of prolonged use of anticonvulsant medication and (2) the presence of an incompletely controlled seizure disorder, usually involving the limbic system, which preceded the development of psychosis.

Reynolds (1971) has emphasized the possibility that anticonvulsant medication may cause epileptic psychosis. He has presented evidence that anticonvulsants often lower serum, red-blood-cell and spinal-fluid-folate levels. He feels that mental changes encountered in epileptics may result from a similar depression of folate and also vitamin B_{12} levels in brain tissue. There is, as yet, no direct evidence that brain levels of these vitamins are lower in psychotic epileptics than nonpsychotic ones, nor is there general agreement that low folate levels in treated epileptics have any relationship to either psychosis or seizure control as postulated by Reynolds (Norris and Pratt, 1971). It is possible that chronic anticonvulsant therapy may have a toxic effect on mental functioning which is mediated by some mechanism other than interaction with folate or B_{12}. Actual drug toxicity does not seem likely to be a major factor in most cases of epileptic psychosis, however, since the amount of medication taken by patients bears little apparent relation to either the incidence or severity of psychosis. Also, it is well known that psychosis may develop even in untreated epileptics (Asuni and Pillutla, 1967).

Other hypotheses to explain the development of epileptic psychosis must be considered. If the psychosis were a form of epilepsy in which the symptoms of schizophrenia were the direct result of epileptic discharges within the brain, a direct correlation might be expected between seizure frequency and the severity of psychosis. If this were so then anticonvulsants would be the treatment of choice for both, but this is usually not the case.

It is also possible that the psychosis is a psychological reaction to years of seizure episodes in which clouded consciousness and periodic sensations of a disturbing nature, often bearing no relation to external reality, lead to confusion of reality with subjective experience. While this mechanism cannot be ruled out in some patients, others with epileptic psychosis have not experienced seizures of this type. Also, the great majority of patients with psychomotor seizures, even those with frequent "twilight states," do not develop psychosis.

On the basis of what is known about the limbic system, it is tempting to hypothesize that the schizophrenialike psychosis of epilepsy is the result of abnormal electrical activity in limbic structures over a number of years which may or may not be associated with frequent clinical convulsions. In this hypothesis psychosis would result from "subictal" or "interictal" discharging lesions in sensitive limbic areas of the brain which would present as atypical psychomotor seizures. The "interictal state" would be the abnormal behavior or thought pattern; the "subictal discharge" would be the abnormal electrical firing, usually in limbic structures, which contributes to or actually causes the interictal state. The psychological correlate of the interictal state has been described as a fluctuating disorder of cerebral functioning with "fluidity of thought processes, loss of trains of associations, word finding difficulties and faulty cognitive functioning" (Glaser et al., 1963; Glaser, 1964). Usually the disorder does not respond to anticonvulsant medication. Sometimes, but not usually, the psychotic disorder may be related to a specific psychological disturbance. The confusion and intellectual disorganization of the psychotic disorder more often develop gradually and seem unrelated to environmental turmoil. Such interictal disturbances are occasionally difficult to distinguish from psychomotor seizures. However, they may persist for days, weeks or months and may not be associated with a clear-cut seizure, although at times they may lead to one. When this is the case a major (grand mal) seizure may seem to clear up the preceding interictal state and the patient may return to a more normal mental condition at least temporarily. During the interictal state the EEG may show unmodified rhythms, desynchronization, disappearance of abnormal discharges or a reinforced temporal abnormality (Glaser, 1964). Recording the EEG from the scalp can be misleading since it may not reveal epileptiform discharges that can be detected simultaneously in the amygdaloid region with depth electrodes (Bickford, 1957).

There is no clear answer to the question of whether subictal discharges can lead to severe abnormality of behavior and thought in patients who have never had a recognizable seizure, although it seems likely that this may occur in both adults (Ervin et al., 1965) and children (Green, 1961). The results of anticonvulsant therapy, however, are usually disappointing when temporal spikes are associated with behavioral abnormality in the absence of seizures.

It is apparent that the relationship of psychosis to epilepsy cannot be easily defined. The prolonged behavioral disturbances which respond to anticonvulsants (Friedlander and Feinstein, 1956; Goldensohn and Gold, 1960) seem to be manifestations of seizures. These include confusion, withdrawal, negativism, fogginess, and hostility.

The use of major tranquilizers such as fluphenazine (an "alerting" phenothiazine) alone or in combination with anticonvulsants appears to be a successful therapeutic approach to patients with an interictal psychosis (Detre and Feldman, 1963; Detre and Jarecki, 1971). Although high or rapidly increasing doses of phenothiazines can precipitate seizures in some patients, low or slowly increasing doses often have a beneficial effect on the psychosis and they sometimes seem to help in diminishing the frequency of a patient's seizures. This is especially so in patients whose seizure frequency appears to be aggravated by anxiety. The treatment of psychosis is purely symptomatic and must proceed on a trial-and-error basis. There are as yet no carefully controlled studies which have established the benefit of ataractic drugs in the treatment of epileptic psychosis.

It may be extremely difficult in an individual case to distinguish ordinary schizophrenia from the schizophrenialike psychosis of epilepsy. In both conditions the psychosis may begin in the second or third decade and the course varies. Remission may occur in either but both tend to be chronic. Though personality and affect tend to be less abnormal in epileptic psychosis, symptomatically the two psychotic conditions may be virtually indistinguishable. However, the family history and a positive medical history of epilepsy provide important information. In ordinary schizophrenia there is a very high incidence of serious psychopathology in the immediate family of affected patients. There is a 10 to 15 per cent chance that first-degree relatives will be diagnosed as schizophrenic. By contrast, the incidence of schizophrenia in the family of patients with epileptic psychosis does not exceed that of the general population (Glithero, Slater, Beard, 1963). A history of epilepsy is, of course, the major distinguishing feature, positive in epileptic psychosis and negative in ordinary schizophrenia. The EEG may be of some help in differential diagnosis as electroencephalographic abnormalities, particularly those implicating the anterior temporal regions, are characteristic of epileptic psychosis. Abnormal EEG's are seen, however, with increased frequency in schizophrenics and normal EEG's are not unusual in epileptic psychotics. Phenothiazines are beneficial but anticonvulsant drugs are of only limited therapeutic usefulness in the two conditions.

SEIZURES AND SEXUAL ACTIVITY

The relationship between abnormal sexual behavior and epilepsy has often been noted but rarely studied. Gastaut and Collomb (1954) reported that hyposexuality existed in two-thirds of 36 temporal lobe epileptics but was infrequent in patients with other types of epilepsy. A striking feature of this hyposexuality was poverty of sexual drive rather than impotence. The condition seemed to follow the onset of seizures. Sexual drive did not develop at all in psychomotor epilepsy beginning in childhood. Sexual interest diminished after the onset of psychomotor epilepsy in adults. A study by Taylor (1969) of 100 psychomotor epileptics before and after temporal lobectomy confirmed the findings of Gastaut and Collomb. Only 14 had a satisfactory adjustment preoperatively. Postoperatively, these 14 remained normal, 22 others had improved, 14 worsened and 50 maintained the same poor adjustment. Those who had improved also experienced the greatest relief from seizures.

A relationship between epilepsy and impotence has also been suggested. Hierons and Saunders (1966) reported 15 cases of impotence unrelated to diminished libido in patients with temporal lobe lesions. It is not clear whether these findings reflect the selection of patients studied or are an accurate representation of the psychosexual adjustment of all patients with temporal lobe epilepsy. It is not uncommon for sexual problems to appear in any chronically ill patient. However, the experimental evidence which relates sexual function to the limbic system provides a further reason to expect some sort of sexual dysfunction in psychomotor epilepsy. Destructive lesions in the amygdala have given rise to indiscriminate hypersexuality (Kluver and Bucy, 1939) and stimulation of limbic structures has given rise to erections (MacLean and Ploog, 1962). "Sexual seizures" have been noted in temporal lobe epileptics but this is quite rare (Currier et al., 1971).

Other studies have suggested a relatively high incidence of various sexual deviations among temporal lobe epileptics (Kolorsky, 1967). As the studies have been far from conclusive, this is not an established clinical fact. Clearly, most sexual deviates do not have seizures. Heightened heterosexual activity appears to be exceedingly rare after the onset of psychomotor seizures.

BEHAVIORAL SIGNIFICANCE OF ABNORMAL EEG's IN THE ABSENCE OF SEIZURES

During the laboratory evaluation of a psychiatric patient it is not uncommon to find an abnormal EEG when there is no evidence of overt seizures. As one might presume, the relationship between an abnormal EEG and behavior disturbance in nonepileptic patients is even more difficult to define than it is in epileptics, primarily because there are major variables which are very difficult to control.

How sure can a clinician be that a patient with a behavior disturbance and an abnormal EEG does not in fact have a seizure disorder? The criteria for such a judgment are almost never ex plicitly stated. Hill (1957) has reported that a high percentage of schizophrenic patients show such paroxysmal abnormalities in their EEG's as synchronous spikes, spike-and-wave complexes (usually in the 4-5 cps range), and slow wave bursts. Some of these patients actually did demonstrate seizures and some of them therefore might have had epileptic psychosis. The criteria which are listed on p. 21 may help to distinguish behavior caused by psychomotor seizures from neurotic or psychotic behavior.

Defining the limits of normality in the EEG is also a major problem. There is no doubt that spikes, spike-wave discharges, focal slowing with phase reversal, and paroxysmal activity during wakefulness are always abnormal. But, there remains a question about theta rhythms intermixed with a dominant alpha pattern, prolonged slowing after hyperventilation or even 14 and 6 positive spikes, all of which are seen so often in normal adolescents. Do these have clinical significance or are they merely maturational deviations from the norm that the individual will outgrow? This question cannot as yet be answered. In patients who drink heavily or who have received tranquilizers or other medications, electroencephalographic abnormalities may represent the effect of these drugs or withdrawal from them (Table 1-2). The electroencephalographic abnormalities seen in some "psychopathic" patients with a history of aggressive behavior may possibly be secondary to brain damage. Hostile behavior often elicits hostile reactions and head injuries are quite commonly sustained during fights by patients who habitually start them. Thus, brain damage and positive electroencephalographic findings in aggressive patients may be the result and not the cause of emotional disturbance. Yet, even with these possibilities in mind there still remains a considerable literature correlating electroencephalographic abnormalities with certain psychiatric symptoms.

In a large series of unselected, nonepileptic psychiatric patients it was possible to differentiate those with abnormal EEG's from those with normal EEG's on the basis of their symptoms (Tucker et al., 1965). Symptoms of a kind classically associated with schizophrenia were significantly more common in the psychiatric patients with abnormal EEG's. These included impaired associations, flattened affect, religiosity, persecutory and somatic delusions, auditory hallucinations, impaired personal habits and destructive-assaultive behavior. The group with abnormal EEG's also exhibited symptoms classically associated with neurological diseases such as time disorientation, perseveration, recent memory difficulty, and headaches. Neurotic and depressed patients had roughly the same incidence of abnormal EEG's as the general population (18 per cent).

The incidence of EEG abnormality among "psychopaths" and children with serious behavior disorders is greater than 50 per cent. In schizophrenia the incidence is 24 per cent to 40 per cent (Ellingson, 1955; Hill, 1963; Williams, 1969). Nevertheless, the diagnosis of brain damage, epilepsy, or psychosis cannot be made on the basis of electroencephalographic criteria alone and the meaning of abnormal recordings in the absence of seizures or clinical symptoms cannot always be determined.

Table 1-3
Effect of Commonly Used Drugs on the EEG*

Drug	*Effect on Basic Frequencies*	EEG Changes Synchronization	*New Waves*	*Persistence after Drug Discontinued*
Phenothiazine	slowing sometimes beta	increased	high voltage sharp	6-10 wks.
Tricyclics	increased beta	increased	sharp	?
Barbiturates	increased beta; slowing	increased in low doses; decreased in high doses	spindles	3-6 wks.
Meprobamate	increased beta	increased	spindles	3-6 wks.
Benzodiazepines	increased beta	increased	Fast, sharp	3-6 wks.

All drugs but barbiturates tend to increase pre-existing dysrhythmias. Withdrawal from high levels of barbiturates and meprobamate can induce increased slowing, synchronization, and paroxysmal activity and may result in seizures.
* Fink, 1963; Ulett et al., 1965

REFERENCES

Asuni, T. and V. S. Pillutla.   Schizophrenia-like psychoses in Nigerian epileptics. Brit. J. Psychiat. 113: 1375, 1967.

Bickford, R. G.   New dimensions in electroencephalography. Neurology 7: 469, 1957.

Bower, B. R. and P. M. Jeavons.   The effect of corticotrophin and prednisolone on infantile spasms with mental retardation. Arch. Dis. Child. 36: 23, 1961.

Bray, P. F. and W. C. Wiser.   Evidence for a genetic etiology of temporal-central abnormalities in focal epilepsy. New Eng. J. Med. 271: 926, 1964.

Chaudry, M. R. and D. A. Pond.   Mental deterioration in epileptic children. J. Neurol. Psychiat. 24: 213, 1961.

Currier, R. D., S. C. Little, J. F. Suess, and O. J. Andy.   Sexual seizures. Arch. Neurol. 25: 260, 1971.

Detre, T. and R. G. Feldman.   Behavior disorder associated with seizure states: pharmacological and psychosocial management. In: G. H. Glaser, ed., EEG and Behavior. Basic Books, New York, p. 366, 1963.

————, and H. G. Jarecki.   Modern Psychiatric Treatment. J. B. Lippincott Co., Philadelphia, 1971.

Ellingson, R. J.   Incidence of EEG abnormality among patients with mental disorders of apparently non organic origin. Critical review. Am. J. Psychiat. 111: 263, 1955.

Ervin, F., A. W. Epstein, and H. E. King.   Behavior of epileptic and nonepileptic patients with "temporal spikes." Arch. Neurol. and Psychiat. 74: 488, 1955.

Fink, M.   Quantitative EEG in human psychopharmacology: drug patterns. In: G. H. Glaser, ed., EEG and Behavior. Basic Books, New York, p. 177, 1963.

Flor-Henry, P.   Psychosis and temporal lobe epilepsy. Epilepsia 10: 363, 1969.

————.   Ictal and interictal psychiatric manifestations in epilepsy: Specific or non-specific? Epilepsia 13:773, 1972.

Friedlander, W. J. and G. H. Feinstein.   Petit mal status: epilepsia minoris continua. Neurology 6: 357, 1956.

Gastaut, H. and H. Collomb.   Étude du comportement sexuel chez les épileptiques psychomoteurs. Ann. Medicopsychol. 112: 657, 1954.

Gibbs, F. A. and E. C. Gibbs.   Atlas of Electroencephalography. Vol. 2. Addison-Wesley Press, Cambridge, Mass., 1952.

Glaser, G. H., R. J. Newman, and R. Schafer. Interictal psychosis in psychomotor temporal lobe epilepsy: an EEG-psychological study. In: G. H. Glaser, ed., EEG and Behavior. Basic Books, New York, p. 345, 1963.

――――. The problem of psychosis in psychomotor temporal lobe epileptics. Epilepsia 5: 271, 1964.

Goldensohn, E. S. and A. P. Gold. Prolonged behavioral disturbances as ictal phenomena. Neurology 10: 1, 1960.

Green, J. B. Association of behavior disorder with electroencephalographic focus in children without seizure. Neurology 11: 337, 1961.

Green, J. D. The hippocampus. Physiol. Rev. 44: 561, 1964.

Guerrant, J., W. W. Anderson, A. Fischer, M. R. Weinstein, R. M. Jaros, and A. Deskins. Personality in Epilepsy. C. C. Thomas, Springfield, Ill., 1962.

Hierons, R. and M. Saunders. Impotence in patients with temporal lobe lesions. Lancet 2: 761, 1966.

Hill, D. Electroencephalogram in schizophrenia. In: D. Richter, ed., Schizophrenia: Somatic Aspects. Pergamon Press, London, p. 33, 1957.

――――. The EEG in psychiatry. In: J. D. N. Hill and G. Parr, eds. Electroencephalography. Macmillan Co., Oxford, p. 368, 1963.

Hunter, J. and H. H. Jasper. Effects of thalamic stimulation in unanesthetized animals: the arrest reaction and petit mal-like seizures, activation patterns and generalized convulsions. EEG Clin. Neurophysiol. 1: 305, 1949.

Inouye, E. Observations on forty twin index cases with chronic epilepsy and their co-twins. J. Nerv. Ment. Dis. 130: 401, 1960.

Kluver, H. and P. C. Bucy. Preliminary analysis of functions of the temporal lobes in monkeys. Arch. Neurol. Psychiat. 42: 979, 1939.

Kolorsky, A., K. Freund, J. Machek, and O. Polak. Male sexual deviation. Arch. Gen. Psychiat. 17: 735, 1967.

Lennox, W. G. The heredity of epilepsy as told by relatives and twins. J.A.M.A. 146: 529, 1951.

Lilienfeld, A. M. and B. Pasamanick. Association of maternal and fetal factors with the development of epilepsy. J.A.M.A. 155: 719, 1954.

MacLean, P. D. and D. W. Ploog. Cerebral representation of penile erection. J. Neurophysiol. 25: 29, 1962.

Marcus, E. M. and C. W. S. Watson. Symmetrical epileptogenic foci in monkey cerebral cortex. Mechanisms of interaction and regional variations in capacity for synchronous discharges. Arch. Neurol. 19: 99, 1968.

Margerison, J. H. and J. Corsellis. Epilepsy and the temporal lobes. Brain 89: 499, 1966.

Marshall, A. G., E. O. Hutchinson, and J. Honisett. Heredity in common diseases: a retrospective survey of twins in a hospital population. Brit. Med. J. 1: 1, 1962.

Metrakos, K. and J. D. Metrakos. Genetics of convulsive disorders: II Genetic and encephalographic studies in centrencephalic epilepsy. Neurology 11: 474, 1961.

Norris, J. W. and R. F. Pratt. A controlled study of folic acid in epilepsy. Neurology 21: 659, 1971.

Ounsted, C., J. Lindsay, and R. Norman. Biological Factors in Temporal Lobe Epilepsy. William Heinemann Medical Books Ltd., London, 1966.

Pond, D. A. Psychiatric aspects of epilepsy. J. Ind. Med. Prof. 3: 1441, 1957.

Posner, J. B., F. Plum, and A. Posnak. Cerebral metabolism during electrically induced seizures in man. Arch. Neurol. 20: 388, 1969.

Reynolds, E. H. Anticonvulsant drugs, folic acid metabolism, fit frequency and psychiatric illness. Psychiat. Neurol. Neurochir. 74: 167, 1971.

Rodin, E. A. The Prognosis of Patients with Epilepsy. C. C. Thomas, Springfield, Ill., 1968.

Slater, E., A. W. Beard, and E. Glithero. The schizophrenia-like psychosis of epilepsy. Brit. J. Psychiat. 109: 95, 1963.

Small, J. G., V. Milstein, and J. R. Stevens. Are psychomotor epileptics different? Arch. Neurol. 7: 187, 1962.

Srole, L., et al. Mental Health in the Metropolis. McGraw-Hill Book Co., New York, 1962.

Taylor, D. C. Sexual behavior and temporal lobe epilepsy. Arch. Neurol. 21: 510, 1969.

Tower, D. The Neurochemistry of Epilepsy: Seizure Mechanisms and their Management. C. C. Thomas, Springfield, Ill., 1960.

Tucker, G. J., T. Detre, M. Harrow, and G. H. Glaser. Behavior and symptoms of psychiatric patients and the electroencephalogram. Arch. Gen. Psychiat. 12: 278, 1965.

Ulett, G. A., A. F. Heusler, and T. J. Word. The effect of psychotropic drugs on the EEG of the chronic psychotic patient. In: W. P. Wilson, ed., Applications of Electroencephalography in Psychiatry: A symposium. Duke Univ. Press, Durham, p. 241, 1965.

Williams, D. Neural factors related to habitual aggression. Brain 92: 503, 1969.

Chapter 2

LIMBIC SYSTEM

The limbic system is a meeting place for the disciplines of psychiatry and neurology. It is, in a way, more of a philosophic concept than a discrete anatomic or physiological system. The term refers to the ring of gray matter and tracts bordering the hemispheres in the medial portions of the brain that play a role in emotions. Phylogenetically, many of the areas designated as the limbic system are among the oldest portions of the cortex; in lower creatures these structures largely subserve smell and have traditionally been called the rhinencephalon. However, as all regions designated "limbic" are not related to olfaction, and other brain regions beside limbic ones play a role in emotional functions, the term "limbic system" has been criticized (Brodal, 1969). Our rationale for continued use of the term "limbic system" rests upon the corresponding results of stimulation and ablation studies demonstrating consistent interrelationships of its various components, the importance of these regions to emotional functioning, and not least to the wide usage of the term by clinicians, physiologists, and anatomists.

It was Papez (1937) who first pointed out that the limbic system is possibly related to emotion, behavior, and visceral reactivity. He regarded the hippocampus as a regulator of hypothalamic centers concerned with emotional responses. On the basis of his observations of patients with rabies (which affects the hippocampus and causes emotional and behavioral changes, such as anxiety and paroxysms of rage and terror), Papez predicted that following stimulation of the limbic system there could be prolonged active discharges in its own structures with very little spread to neocortical areas because of the interconnections between the limbic system structures. He predicted that these "reverberating circuits" of discharge within the limbic system would produce marked alterations in the subjective emotional life of an individual. In effect, Papez proposed an anatomic and physiologic substrate for intense affective reactions and instincts which are customarily the domain of much psychiatric theory and research.

At the time Papez published his paper on the limbic system, Freudian theory was in wide vogue. The idea of a phylogenetically ancient, deep, central portion of the nervous system which influenced behavior and thought not under conscious, neocortical control was consistent with some Freudian concepts of instinctual drive. The reasoning went something like this: The sense of smell in lower animals seems to be closely associated with memory, instinct, and emotion, for it is often smell which alerts an animal to danger and provokes fear, flight, or fighting, as well as sexual arousal and mating. Smell and memory in such animals must be related functions as it is important for lower animals to remember the associations of particular smells. The autonomic nervous system must be closely related to the rhinencephalon since such autonomic responses as pupillary dilatation, piloerection, increased heart rate and blood flow to skeletal muscles occur in response to environmental circumstances in which an animal must fight or flee or prepare for mating. While the sense of smell is no longer as important to human life, it is postulated that these rhinencephalic structures and the limbic system in man are still involved with emotions, memory, and visceral responses and that disturbances of the limbic system disrupt them.

ANATOMY

The gray-matter structures encompassed by the term "limbic system" include those which are located in the anterior and medial portions of the temporal lobe and those outside the temporal lobe. Many portions of this system in the temporal lobe have separate names such as the amygdala, hippocampus (both the gyrus hippocampus and its medial portion, the hippocampal formation, which is sometimes called Ammon's horn), and the uncus. Limbic structures which are located outside the temporal lobe include the mammilary bodies, anterior nucleus of the thalamus, gyrus cingulus, nuclei of the septum, portions of the midbrain tegmentum (interpeduncular nucleus, lateral midbrain area of Nauta, central gray and ventral tegmental nucleus of Gudden), habenula, subcallosal and supracallosal gyri. The major tracts interconnecting these regions include the fimbria, fornix, mamillothalamic tract,

FIG.2-1

THE LIMBIC SYSTEM

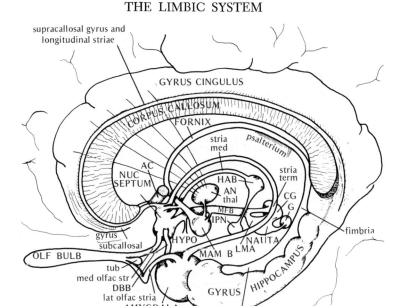

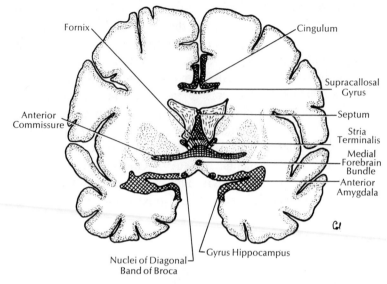

FIG. 2-2A

THE LIMBIC SYSTEM: ANTERIOR CORONAL SECTION

anterior commissure, stria terminalis, stria medullaris, median fore-brain bundle, and diagonal band of Broca (*see Fig. 2-1, 2-2A, 2-2B*).

In order to conceptualize these structures it may be helpful to recall that many of the medial structures of the brain have the shape of a large C, with one end in the anterior temporal lobe and the other in or near the septal region. Among the limbic structures that have this form are: (1) the gyrus cingulus, (2) the fimbria-fornix-mammilary body pathway; (3) the stria terminalis which connects the amygdala and the septal area; and (4) the supracallosal gyrus and longitudinal striae which connect the hippocampus region with the septal region. Other tracts with a curved shape are the median forebrain bundle which connects the septal nuclei with the midbrain tegmentum and the stria medullaris which connects the septal region with the habenula (*Fig.* 2-1). The anterior commissure is a tract which laterally connects the right and left amygdala. The diagonal band of Broca also runs laterally to connect the septum with the amygdala. The tracts which connect the gray matter of the limbic system generally contain both afferent and efferent fibers (*Figs.* 2-1, 2-2A, 2-2B).

The richness of interconnections amongst regions of the limbic system can only partly be appreciated by the account above, and actually not all of the interconnections are known. Each amygdaloid nucleus appears to have direct connections, most of which are reciprocal, with the other amygdaloid nucleus, the olfactory bulb, the septal nuclei, hypothalamus, thalamus, habenula, midbrain, and hippocampus. The hippocampus has connections with

FIG. 2-2B

THE LIMBIC SYSTEM: POSTERIOR CORONAL SECTION

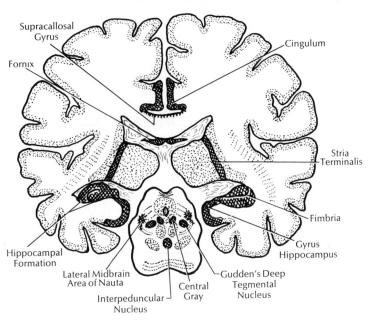

the mammilary bodies, anterior thalamic nucleus, gyrus cingulus, septum, midbrain regions, and amygdala.

PHYSIOLOGICAL PSYCHOLOGY

Efforts to determine the function of the various components of the limbic system have utilized stimulation and ablation studies in animals and to some extent in man. These have yielded evidence that limbic structures influence memory, learning, emotional states (including anxiety, rage, placidity, and alertness), visceral and endocrine responses, and behavior, particularly aggressive, oral, and sexual activity. It is not possible to define the function of each of the parts of the limbic system because none of them acts as a center for a particular function. All portions of the limbic system are more or less associated with all of the functions enumerated above. As Papez predicted, there is a strong tendency after stimulation of limbic structures for prolonged afterdischarges to occur which spread throughout the limbic system with comparatively little involvement of the neocortex (MacLean, 1952, 1954).

The specific aspects of behavior demonstrated by stimulation and ablation studies in the limbic system are of great theoretical interest to both psychiatrists and neurologists, for the behavioral and cognitive alterations produced by experiments in animals closely resemble human responses that are so often considered to be "functional." Stimulation of the hippocampus of cats results in apparent bewilderment and anxiety together with intense attention to something the animal seems to sense in the environment. Such phenomena have been considered alerting and defensive reactions, resulting perhaps from hallucinations induced by the stimulation. Amygdalar stimulation may result in similar reactions.

Bilateral hippocampal destruction leads to recent memory loss with prevention of new learning in both animals and man. Destruction of other portions of the limbic system also produces deficits in recent memory. Bilateral ablation of the anterior gyrus cingulus and bilateral division of the fornices have resulted in similar deficits.

Stimulation of portions of the amygdala results in rage reactions in animals. Similar reactions have been seen after stimulation of the midbrain gray matter or the placement of destructive lesions in the septum. Stimulation of the amygdala in animals has provoked reactions that have been interpreted as reflecting feelings of fear. Sensations of fear have also been described in conscious human beings while this region was stimulated during surgery. Chewing, gagging, licking, retching, swallowing, bladder contractions, respiratory, pulse, and blood pressure increases, and increased secretion of ACTH have all been produced by amygdalar stimulation as well as stimulation elsewhere in the limbic brain. Such phenomena are quite similar to the manifestations of psychomotor epilepsy. This clinical similarity and the characteristic anterior temporal spikes seen in the EEG of patients with psychomotor epilepsy led some clinicians to apply the term "limbic epilepsy" to such seizures (Fulton, 1952).

The bizarre behavioral alterations (e.g., docility, loss of natural fear, compulsive oral activity, and heightened indiscriminate sexual activity) noted by Kluver and Bucy (1939) after bilateral removal of the amygdaloid nuclei and overlying hippocamal cortex provided further evidence for the limbic system's role in these functions. Similar changes have been noted in man after bilateral temporal lobectomies which, if performed somewhat caudal to the amygdala, also produce profound memory loss, particularly for recent events.

Considering the relationship between the limbic system and emotions, it might be predicted that diseases involving limbic structures would cause emotional disorders. This does seem to be the case in psychomotor-temporal lobe epilepsy, as noted above. It also seems to be so in other conditions which involve limbic structures.

Malamud (1967) studied 18 patients with intracranial neoplasms which involved limbic structures. All had originally been diagnosed as having psychiatric disorders. Ten were thought to be schizophrenics, four were depressed, one was manic, and the others appeared severely neurotic. Eleven of the patients had psychomotor seizures.

Subacute and chronic forms of viral encephalitis tend to affect the medial portions of the temporal lobes, which are associated with the limbic system (Glaser and Pincus, 1969; Himmelhoch et al., 1970). Such forms of viral encephalitis characteristically give rise to behavioral symptoms which are often suggestive of psychiatric disorders. Early in the course of subacute encephalitis, this may be the cause of diagnostic confusion; the disease has commonly been mistaken for schizophrenia, hysteria, or depression. The behavioral alterations seen in these patients probably are the result of both irritation and destruction of limbic structures.

Gibbs (1951) found that psychiatric disorders were three times more common in patients with anterior temporal seizure foci than in those with seizure foci located elsewhere in the brain.

In patients being examined for epilepsy, electrical stimulation of the amygdala and the hippocampus after placement of chronic electrodes has produced brief alterations which mimic psychomotor seizures and persist only during the passage of current and the limited after-discharge (Stevens et al., 1969). After such stimulation, however, mood and thought disturbances of psychotic proportions may persist for hours.

LIMBIC SYSTEM AND VIOLENT BEHAVIOR
Experimental Background

Experiments on animals and a large accumulation of data on human beings have indicated that violence may be a symptom of a disturbance of brain function. Since Bard's experiments in 1928 it has been clear that brain lesions, decortication, and lesions in the region of the hypothalamus can produce marked alterations in emotional reactivity. Rage reactions in cats which include arching of the back, piloerection, snarling, biting, and scratching are seen when the entire cortex, basal ganglia, and most of the thalamus have been removed. The rage phenomena of decorticate cats are directed responses to a variety of environmental stimuli which do not elicit rage reactions in the normal animal. It has been assumed that the decorticate animal is not capable of subjective emotion and accordingly the reaction described above has been called "sham rage." However, this assumption that subjective emotion is a function of portions of the nervous system that had been removed in such animals may not be entirely justified, and it would be a mistake to make too much of the distinction between visible emotional reaction and subjective feeling on the basis of present information.

Removal of the neocortex, leaving the hippocampus, amygdala, hypothalamus, and brain stem intact, does not change the basic personality of the cat. It purrs and responds to affection. However, tail pinching or other stimuli which might elicit mild manifestations of anger in the normal cat, will in the decorticate animal lead to a ferocious, directed attack. Destruction of the ventral medial nucleus of the hypothalamus has produced permanently ferocious animals. Stimulation of portions of the amygdala, posterior hypothalamus, or midbrain also may enhance aggressive hunting behavior in which the animal will go to great lengths to make an attack upon some object it would normally avoid or ignore such as a larger animal or a toy. Stimulation of other portions of the limbic system may stop attack behavior, and bilateral amygdalectomy makes ferocious animals permanently placid (Kluver and Bucy, 1939); yet, occasionally, the reverse has been reported.

Placid, amygdalectomized animals can be made fierce by producing lesions of the ventral medial nucleus of the hypothalamus. Rats made savage by lesions in the septal region can be tranquilized by an amygdalectomy. Violent behavior in cats, monkeys, and humans may result from the electrical stimulation of several portions of the limbic system. Destruction of these regions or stimulation of other limbic regions can inhibit such behavior (Mark and Ervin, 1970).

The evidence from animal experiments suggesting a relationship between the neocortex, limbic system, and brain stem and violence is voluminous. Many of the observations and experiments have been contradictory and one may select evidence from them to support almost any reasonable argument. It seems likely that the complex actions and subjective feelings involved in violent aggressiveness must be mediated by extensive collaboration among many parts of the brain (Brodal, 1969). It remains clear, however, that stimulation or destruction of discrete structures within the nervous system can lead to marked alterations in behavior ranging from violence to placidity. It is also clear that the amygdala, hippocampus, and other limbic structures are particularly sensitive in this regard.

VIOLENCE IN MAN

Despite the accumulation of research data linking violence to brain dysfunction, not enough is presently known about human violence to justify a dogmatic categorization. While violence may be a manifestation of brain dysfunction, it is certainly manifested by individuals who are otherwise ostensibly normal. For example, there is no evidence of brain abnormality in most dyssocial individuals nor in those whose violence is limited to an isolated instance of provoked attack. By dyssocial individuals we mean criminals who are like ordinary citizens and are motivated to gain but through illegal means. The Mafia may exemplify this group.

Episodic Violence

If one excludes from consideration dyssocial individuals and those rare cases of repeated violence committed by patients with demonstrable epilepsy or psychosis and concentrates on the remaining group of individuals who display repeatedly violent behavior provoked by minimal stimuli certain remarkably constant features may be found. The group is largely composed of young men from disrupted families who show some evidence of neurologic dysfunction and who often have an unusual susceptibility to alcohol.

Clinical Features

Males predominate by as much as 9:1. The propensity for violence begins in early childhood, lasts through adolescence and the third decade, but declines in at least 40 per cent of cases in the fourth decade (Robins, 1966). So consistently does the history of violence in these people extend back to the preschool and elementary school years that in those cases in which violence first begins after puberty, there must be a strong suspicion that a psychosis or identifiable brain disease has developed (Detre et al., 1972).

EEG abnormalities are quite prevalent in this group. In a study of 1250 individuals in jail for crimes of aggression, Williams (1969) found abnormal EEG's in 57 per cent of the habitual aggressors and in only 12 per cent of those who had committed a solitary aggressive crime, after prisoners who were mentally retarded, epileptic, or had sustained serious head injury were separated from the group. Of the habitual aggressors who had electroencephalographic abnormalities, the temporal lobe was involved in over 80 per cent.

In a study of more than 400 violent prisoners in a large penitentiary, it was discovered that half had symptoms suggestive of epileptic phenomena, one-third had abnormal EEG's, but fewer than 10 per cent had frank temporal lobe epilepsy (Mark and Ervin, 1970). It was also apparent that these people had a characteristic social history which included multiple physical assaults, aggressive sexual behavior including attempted rape, many traffic violations, serious automobile accidents, and a peculiar susceptibility to alcohol called "pathological intoxication."

Effect of Alcohol

Alcohol is one of the few drugs known to precipitate or worsen episodes of violence in individuals with a past history of violent behavior (Guze and Cartwell, 1965; Detre et al., 1972). The state of pathological intoxication is not synonymous with ordinary drunkenness. The term refers to a state in which the individual engages in a violent act after drinking, an act for which he will have little or no recollection. Such behavior may sometimes be elicited by small amounts of alcohol, much less than would be required for ordinary intoxication. Blood alcohol levels below 30 mg per 100 ml have been recorded in these cases. Pathological intoxication is not associated with slurred speech and incoordination and may last for only a few minutes. It occurs most often when alcohol is imbibed under circumstances "conducive" to violence, i.e., at a bar or a party, and it has been difficult to reproduce this state of intoxication by administering alcohol in any quantity in a laboratory setting or by intravenous injection. Those who become pathologically intoxicated may not be chronic alcoholics and the condition is not limited to individuals with a criminal disposition. It is relatively rare, even amongst brain-damaged individuals. Yet 90 per cent of pathological-intoxication cases are associated with brain damage, epilepsy, retardation, or psychosis (Bowman and Jellinck, 1941). Electroencephalographic changes may also be associated with episodes of pathological intoxication (Thompson, 1963). There is clearly an interplay between environmental and organic factors in the induction of pathological intoxication which, if understood, might shed light on the complex relationship between brain dysfunction and violence.

Etiology

It is likely that the "dyscontrol syndrome" described by Mark and Ervin is the same syndrome that Detre calls "explosive personality disorder" and that others have termed "impulsive neurosis" or "criminal sociopathic personality." The combination of a characteristic past history of violent behavior with commonly associated electroencephalographic abnormalities which often involve the temporal lobe certainly suggests that the antisocial behavior may be determined by neurological, if not by limbic, abnormality.

Some studies have suggested that habitual acts of antisocial behavior involving physical violence are genetically determined. While the point remains very controversial, it appears that XYY chromosomes may be associated with tall stature and aggressiveness (Hook and Kim, 1970; Jacobs et al., 1971). Twin studies have indicated that concordance rates for delinquency are higher in monozygotic than in dizygotic twin pairs; however, such evidence for a genetic influence in episodically violent behavior is not entirely conclusive (Slater and Cowie, 1971), and the dominant view today is that an unfavorable environment in childhood is the major determining factor in episodic violence.

There is considerable evidence that associates a disruption of family life with the development of episodic violence. Troubled family life including brutality, alcoholism, and marital discord is such a constant feature in the background of repeatedly violent persons that it is possible to predict the development of delinquent behavior with great accuracy on the basis of certain personality and family factors. When all of the five following factors are found in two- to three-year-old children, it seems likely that delinquency can be predicted with the same degree of accuracy (90 per cent) as it can in five- and six-year-olds (Glueck and Glueck, 1966): (1) psychopathology of either or both parents (alcoholism, delinquency, emotional disturbance, or mental retardation); (2) indifference or hostility to the child on the part of one or both parents; (3) extreme restlessness in the child; (4) nonsubmissiveness of the child to parental authority; (5) unusual destructiveness in the child.

On the basis of this association, however, it would be a mistake to attribute violence in the offspring to purely environmental factors since brutality, alcoholism, and marital discord in parents may themselves be expressions of a genetic defect in their personalities. There is support for this contention in Heston's report (1966) that criminality and other associated sociopathic disorders were significantly more prevalent in the offspring of schizophrenics raised in foster homes than in the offspring of nonschizophrenics who were also raised in foster homes. Another possible factor to be considered in the association of environmental stress and violence is the effect of a violent juvenile delinquent upon his parents. The child's problem may be so severe that it disrupts the life of the whole family (Bell, 1968).

On the basis of present evidence it is not possible to determine whether "nurture" or "nature" is more important in the development of episodic violent behavior. What does seem clear, however, is that episodic violence is not a simple functional psychological disorder. Neurologic factors are clearly present and the syndrome cannot be reversed by any known therapeutic means. To the extent that episodic violence is a learned behavioral pattern, it is one that is learned at a very early age (Detre et al., 1972). It appears to be at least as difficult to alter episodic violence in the adult human being as it is to alter the abnormal socialization of adult monkeys which results from social deprivation early in life (Harlow, 1971).

Treatment

Anticonvulsants and antipsychotic drugs are seldom effective in nonepileptic, nonpsychotic offenders in reducing violence. Psychosurgery involving stimulation or ablation of portions of the limbic system, as described by Mark and Ervin (1970), is ethically controversial and would appear to be of limited clinical applicability. Psychotherapy and environmental therapy also seem to be of limited usefulness. In a study of treated juvenile delinquents (one-third of whom were violent) at a well-organized residential center, 75 per cent were found to have had two or more re-convictions after discharge (Hartelius, 1965). Roughly the same rate of recidivism has been noted in other populations of untreated violent criminals (Gibbins et al., 1959).

Unfortunately, the question of how to treat episodic violence is largely academic. Most often violent individuals are presented to neurologists and psychiatrists not as patients but as prisoners. Physicians are not usually asked what treatment will prevent future violence but rather what is the extent of the individual's responsibility for his past violent behavior.

The legal system generally operates under the presumption of unfettered free will. People are assumed to be responsible for their actions. The law recognizes, however, that the operation of free will in certain circumstances is constrained by disease of the brain. Accordingly, the M'Naughten rule and the irresistible impulse rule have been developed and the plea of temporary insanity has become conventional. Attorneys for defendants charged with serious crimes commonly seek to prove that their client's responsibility for his actions was significantly diminished when the crimes occurred. Psychosis, epilepsy, and mental retardation have been established as "a way out" for some accused individuals. In our opinion, the preponderance of evidence does indicate that episodic violence can be a behavioral syndrome which is as organically determined as schizophrenia or epilepsy. Since, however, the best predictor of violent, aggressive behavior in the future is a history of violent or aggressive behavior in the past and since the tendency to recidivism persists at least until the fourth decade of life, it would seem reasonable to separate such individuals from society in some manner until they reach the fourth decade or until some truly effective therapeutic measure is developed.

REFERENCES

Bard, P. A diencephalic mechanism for the expression of rage with special reference to the sympathetic nervous system. Am. J. Physiol. 84: 490, 1928.

Bell, R. Q. A reinterpretation of the direction of effects in studies of socialization. Psychol. Rev. 75: 81, 1968.

Bowman, K. M. and E. M. Jellinck. Alcoholic mental disorders. Quart. J. Stud. Alc. 2: 312, 1941.

Brodal, A. Neurological Anatomy in Relation to Clinical Medicine. 2nd ed. Oxford University Press, New York, 1969.

Detre, T. P., D. J. Kupfer, and S. Taub. The Nosology of Violence: Presentation at Neurological Symposium on the Neural Basis of Violence and Aggression. Houston, Texas, March 1972.

————, and H. G. Jarecki. Modern Psychiatric Treatment. J. B. Lippincott Co., Philadelphia, 1971.

Fulton, H. H. Discussion. Epilepsia 2: 77, 1953.

Gibbens, T. C. N., D. A. Pond, and D. Stafford-Clark. Followup study of criminal psychopaths. J. Ment. Sci. 105: 108, 1959.

Gibbs, F. A. Ictal and nonictal psychiatric disorders in temporal lobe epilepsy. J. Nerv. Ment. Dis. 113: 522, 1951.

Glaser, G. H. and J. H. Pincus. Limbic encephalitis. J. Nerv. Ment. Dis. 149: 59, 1969.

Glueck, E. T. and S. Glueck. Identification of potential delinquents at 2-3 years of age. Int. J. Soc. Psychiat. 12: 5, 1966.

Guerrant, J., W. W. Anderson, A. Fischer, A. Weinstein, R. M. Jaros, and A. Deskins. Personality in Epilepsy. C. C. Thomas, Springfield, Ill., 1962.

Guze, S. B. and D. P. Cartwell. Alcoholism, parole observations and criminal recidivism; study of 116 parolees. Am. J. Psychiat. 122: 436, 1965.

Harlow, H. F., M. K. Harlow, and S. J. Suomi. From thought to therapy: lessons from a primate laboratory. How investigation of the learning capabilities of rhesus monkeys has led to the study of their behavioral abnormalities and rehabilitation. Am. Scien. 59: 538, 1971.

Hartelius, H. Study of male juvenile delinquency. Acta. Psychiat. Scand. 40: 7, 1965.

Heston, L. L. Psychiatric disorders in foster home reared children of schizophrenic mothers. Brit. J. Psychiat. 112: 819, 1966.

Himmelhoch, J., J. H. Pincus, G. J. Tucker, and T. P. Detre. Subacute encephalitis: behavioral and neurological aspects. Brit. J. Psychiat. 116: 531, 1970.

Hook, E. B. and D. S. Kim. Prevalence of XYY and XXY karyotypes in 337 non-retarded young offenders. New Eng. J. Med. 283: 410, 1970.

Jacobs, P. A., W. H. Prince, S. Richmond, and R. A. W. Ratecliff.

Chromosome surveys in penal institutions and approved schools. J. Med. Genet. 8: 49, 1971.

Kluver, H. and P. C. Bucy. Preliminary analysis of functions of the temporal lobes in monkeys. Arch. Neurol. Psychiat. 42: 979, 1939.

MacLean, P. D. Some psychiatric implications of physiological studies on fronto temporal portion of limbic system (visceral brain). Electroenceph. Clin. Neurophysiol. 4: 407, 1952.

MacLean, P. D. The limbic system and its hippocampal formation. Studies in animals and their possible relation to man. J. Neurosurg. 11: 29, 1954.

Malamud, N. Psychiatric disorder with intracranial tumors of the limbic system. Arch. Neurol. 17: 113, 1967.

Mark, V. H. and F. R. Ervin. Violence and the Brain. Harper & Row, New York, 1970.

Papez, J. W. A proposed mechanism of emotion. Arch. Neurol. Psychiat. 38: 725, 1937.

Robins, L. N. Deviant Children Grown Up: Sociological and Psychiatric Study of Sociopathic Personality. Williams & Wilkins, Baltimore, 1966.

Slater, E. and V. Cowie. The Genetics of Mental Disorders. Oxford University Press, London, 1971.

Small, J. G., V. Milstein, and J. R. Stevens. Are psychomotor epileptics different? Arch. Neurol. 7: 187, 1962.

Stevens, J. R. Psychiatric implications of psychomotor epilepsy. Arch. Gen. Psychiat. 14: 461, 1966.

Stevens, J. R., V. H. Mark, F. Erwin, P. Pacheco, and K. Suematsu. Deep temporal stimulation in man: long latency, long lasting psychological changes. Arch. Neurol. 21: 157, 1969.

Thompson, G. N. Electroencephalogram in acute pathological alcoholic intoxication. Bull. Los Ang. Neurol. Soc. 28: 217, 1963.

Williams, D. Neurol factors related to habitual aggression. Brain 92: 503, 1969.

Chapter 3

SCHIZOPHRENIA

Schizophrenia, manifested most notably by bizarre or delusional thoughts, is often easier to diagnose than to define. Nonetheless, on the basis of a distinctive and consistent constellation of symptoms and elements in the family history, it must be considered a dysfunction of the central nervous system. The consistency of these symptoms lends support to the disease concept of schizophrenia for the clinical picture has changed little in time and varies only slightly from culture to culture (Sanua, 1969). The means of establishing the diagnosis of schizophrenia are limited exclusively to history and observation, particularly the age of onset, the clinical course, the characteristically abnormal family history, and the phenomenology of the symptoms as well as the response to treatment. At present there are no laboratory examinations that can establish the diagnosis. Largely for this reason, schizophrenia has been regarded by many clinicians as a functional disorder, the product of environmental stress. In this chapter we will present the criteria that are most helpful in establishing the diagnosis of schizophrenia and differentiating it from other conditions, and we will summarize the evidence that it is an organic dysfunction of the brain.

CLINICAL FEATURES
Age at Onset

Schizophrenia is primarily a disease of young people. Kraeplin noted that most patients were under the age of thirty-five years at the time of diagnosis, a finding which has been confirmed in many subsequent studies. The first clear-cut symptoms appear before the age of twenty-five in 50 per cent of the cases; onset after the age of forty is unusual (Kraepelin, 1925). Symptoms rarely begin in the first decade, but when they do, they virtually always occur in the latter half, never before the age of five. Childhood schizophrenia has often been confused with infantile autism, a condition which usually begins in the first year of life and always appears before age five (see p. 124).

Symptoms

While the criteria put forward by different authors for establishing the diagnosis of schizophrenia vary somewhat, Beck et al. (1962) and Hordern et al. (1968) have found over 80 per cent agreement regarding those cases in which experienced clinicians state that they are positive of the diagnosis. One reason for the differences in the diagnostic criteria has been the attempt to identify a basic symptom or defect in schizophrenic thinking to which all other symptoms are secondary, thus validating a specific etiologic theory of schizophrenia. Yet, if one examines Table 3-1, it is evident that there is actually great consistency among different authors in enumerating the symptoms of schizophrenia and that the differences relate mainly to the emphasis placed upon them individually. Take, for example, the emphasis placed on delusions and hallucinations. Kurt Schneider claimed that if an individual were experiencing any hallucinations or delusions in the absence of disturbances of memory or orientation, or similar symptoms usually associated with delirium or toxic conditions, one could make a decisive clinical diagnosis of schizophrenia (Schneider, 1959). (Table 1) He considered these experiences to be unique to schizophrenia. Despite the importance Schneider attached to delusions and hallucinations, Bleuler regarded them as secondary and instead emphasized loose associations (Bleuler, 1950).

In addition to shifts in emphasis, there are some more substan-

Table 3-1

Summary of Diagnostic and Phenomenological Symptoms
and Signs of Schizophrenia

First Rank Symptoms
(Schneider) (only one necessary for diagnosis)
1. *Auditory Hallucinations*
    a. Audible thoughts (voices speaking patient's thoughts aloud)
    b. Voices arguing (two or more voices arguing usually about patient—refer to patient in third person)
    c. Voices commenting on patient's actions
2. *Delusional Experiences*
    a. Bodily sensations imposed on patient by some external source
    b. Thoughts being taken from his mind
    c. Thoughts ascribed to others
    d. Diffusion of thoughts (patient's thoughts experienced as all around him)
    e. Feelings, impulses, volitional acts imposed on him or under the control of external sources
3. *Delusional Perception* (private meaning of a consensually validated perception)

Diagnostic and Statistical Manual of Mental Disorders

APA, 2nd Ed. (unclear how many necessary for diagnosis)

1. *Disturbances in Thinking*—marked by alterations of Concept formulation leading to misinterpretation of reality and sometimes Delusions and Hallucinations
2. *Mood changes* including ambivalent, constricted, and inappropriate emotional responsiveness and loss of empathy
3. *Behavior* which is withdrawn and regressive and bizarre

Bleuler's Criteria

(Only fundamental necessary)
1. *Fundamental Symptoms*
    a. Loose associations
    b. Impaired affect
    c. Ambivalence
    d. Autism
2. *Intact Functions*
    a. Sensation and perception
    b. Orientation

   c. Memory
   d. Consciousness
   e. Motility
3. *Accessory or Secondary Symptoms*
   a. Hallucinations and delusion
   b. Catatonia
   c. Depressive symptoms

Diagnostic Criteria for Psychiatric Research

(Feighner et al.) (All necessary for diagnosis)
   1. Chronic illness of at least 6 months' duration
   2. Absences of depressive or manic symptoms
   3. Delusions or hallucinations
   4. Verbal productions that make communication difficult because of lack of logical or understandable organization
   5. At least three of the following:
      a. single
      b. poor premorbid social or work adjustment
      c. family history of schizophrenia
      d. absence of alcoholism or drug abuse
      e. onset of illness under age forty

tial differences among the diagnostic schemes listed in Table 3-1. Depression is considered a secondary symptom by Bleuler, yet it rules out the diagnosis according to Feighner, and is not mentioned by Schneider or the American Psychiatric Association (APA, 1968). Feighner's criteria are detailed and clearly useful for research but perhaps too restricted for clinical purposes (Feighner et al., 1972). The APA's scheme is more inclusive but too vague: it justifies the diagnosis of schizophrenia in patients with minimal disorder of thinking and marked mood disturbance. Consequently, the diagnosis of schizophrenia is made more freely in America than in Europe (Hordern et al., 1968). Schneider's criteria for diagnosis, used widely in England, have the advantage of not needing gradation; they are either present or absent. But the symptoms on which it rests are neither unique nor, in our opinion, universally found in schizophrenia. Bleuler's major criteria cannot be easily quantitated. It is not clear how many of the fundamental criteria are necessary for diagnosis or how much of each symptom is indicative of the presence of schizophrenia; hence the relative importance of the symptoms for diagnosis cannot be precisely assessed.

We believe that the most important criteria for establishing the diagnosis of schizophrenia are:

1. A thought disorder characterized by: (a) hallucinations or delusions in the absence of any known cause of these symptoms such as encephalitis, hallucinogenic drugs, or epilepsy; and/or (b) some other form of conceptual disorganization.
2. An early onset of symptoms, usually in young adult life.
3. Absence of major affective symptoms.
4. Absence of major neurological deficits.
5. A progressively deteriorating course of illness or an intermittent course with remissions.
6. A history of schizophrenia in close relatives is useful but not necessary for the diagnosis.

In most classificatory schemes of schizophrenia thought disturbance is considered a basic symptom of schizophrenia. While all patients may not manifest a specific type of thought disorder at all times, some defect in cognition must be present during the course of the illness. It is not difficult to recognize delusions and hallucinations, but conceptual disorganization is a less precise, more inclusive term.

LOOSE ASSOCIATIONS are in Bleuler's view the basis for establishing a diagnosis of schizophrenia. Loosening of associations means an absence of normal connections between expressed thoughts. An overt example of this was given by Bleuler (1950). "My last teacher in that subject was Professor A. He was a man with black eyes. I also like black eyes. There are also blue and gray eyes and other sorts too. I have heard it said that snakes have green eyes. All people have eyes" (Bleuler, 1950, p. 17). In a milder form the patient's thought pattern may not immediately appear to be abnormal, but after 10 or 15 minutes' conversation one may not be quite sure what he is talking about or how he arrived at a particular point. If the examiner then pays attention to the associative pattern he will find that the patient is constantly switching from one topic to another, often introducing new ideas that are unrelated to what has gone before.

Another abnormal pattern of thought that has been characterized as "basic" to schizophrenia is OVERINCLUSION. This refers to the patient's apparent failure to exclude from his consciousness competing, contradictory, or merely irrelevant thoughts so that his thinking is encumbered with ideas which have insufficient connection to his main train of thought (Cameron, 1963). Overinclusion, in our view, can be placed under the rubric of loose association.

Another defect in the thought patterns of schizophrenics has been described in what can be called the ABSTRACT-CONCRETE DIMENSION. The Russian psychologist Vygotsky felt that schizophrenic thought disorder essentially represented loss of the ability to think abstractly and a tendency to concreteness (Vygotsky, 1962). Concreteness has been defined as an attitude which is determined by and cannot proceed beyond some immediate experience, object, or stimulus (Mayer-Gross et al., 1969). From his work on patients with organic brain injuries, Kurt Goldstein developed a similar concept of the "concrete attitude" which he applied to the problem of schizophrenic thinking. Goldstein believed that many of the peculiarities in the behavior of schizophrenics became understandable when considered as an expression of abnormal concreteness (Goldstein, 1944). He was quick to point out, however, that the level and type of concreteness is not identical with that of neurological cases, primarily because of the intrusion of idiosyncratic and personalized ideas in schizophrenic thinking (Goldstein, 1958). (See below.) Not all schizophrenics seem to be concrete or literal and some patients, especially those with markedly paranoid features, have even been described as overly abstract.

A defect that many psychoanalysts consider basic to schizophrenia is found in the *symbolic-logical dimension*. Schizophrenics are seen as "paralogical"; they equate the identities of subjects on the basis of identical predicates, i.e., "I am a woman, the Virgin Mary was a woman, therefore I am Mary" (Von Domarus, 1944). This position is supported by other prominent clinicians such as Arieti (1955). Many of the psychoanalytic interpretations of schizophrenic language emphasize its symbolical, dreamlike nature (Sullivan, 1953).

Among the most striking of the abnormalities of thought and speech in schizophrenics is the idiosyncratic, personalized, and often bizarre character of their verbal expressions (Harrow et al., 1972). When bizarre, this quality is easily noticed, but it may be subtle and may become apparent only during a formal mental status examination. The part of the examination that is especially useful for this purpose is proverb interpretation and the discernment of similarities and differences. For example, when asked the meaning of "People in glass houses should not throw stones," one of our patients replied, "Because people would see me in my house and throw stones at me." Another, when asked what is similar about an apple and an orange, said, "An apple is round and symbolizes perfection but none of us can be perfect." In these responses one can see aspects of many of the disturbances of thinking mentioned above. With the mental status examination one can determine not only personalized, bizarre, and idiosyncratic concept formation in schizophrenics but also abnormal concreteness, loose associations, and overinclusive thought. Obviously, there is much overlap in these descriptions of schizophrenic thought patterns. When examining for schizophrenia it is important to use several proverbs and similarities since abnormal responses may occur only after several adequate answers. Disjointedness, idiosyncracy, and bizarreness seem to be more characteristic of schizophrenia than of any other psychiatric or neurologic condition. If this type of thinking is present one must suspect schizophrenia.

The other "fundamental" symptoms in Bleuler's classification—disturbances of affect, ambivalence, and autism—can be helpful

but are not essential in making a diagnosis of schizophrenia. AF-
FECT in schizophrenics is classically described as "flattened": emotional expression is absent or its range is limited. This is found to
be true more frequently in chronic patients; and in acute schizophrenic breaks it is uncommon. The affect may also be "inappropriate" in that a patient can tell a happy story and appear sad, or
vice versa.

AMBIVALENCE refers to the capacity of schizophrenic patients to
feel intense contradictory emotions at the same time, for instance,
to express both hate and love for a person in almost the same
breath: "I hate that Dr. X and want to strangle him, that wonder-
ful man who saved my life." Neither ambivalence nor flattened
affect is consistently present in schizophrenia; therefore we do not
feel that they are necessary for diagnosis.

Bleuler defined AUTISM as a break with external reality that leads
the patient to become preoccupied with his inner life; this results in an incapacity to develop meaningful human relationships.
External events may become so blended with subjective feelings or
fantasy that the patient sees them as relating specifically to him; at
this point such symptoms could be called delusional or hallucinatory. Autism in schizophrenics appears to be a behavioral result of
thought disorder.

SUBTYPES OF SCHIZOPHRENIA AND PROGNOSIS

The classical diagnostic subtypes of schizophrenia (hebephrenic,
catatonic, undifferentiated, etc.) as delineated in the diagnostic
and statistical nomenclature of the American Psychiatric Association are of little value in ascertaining prognosis or choosing therapy. Phenomenologically, they merely mean that one or the other
of Bleuler's secondary symptoms is prominent. These classical subtypes thus have little more than historical interest. A more recent
distinction of "process" from "reactive" schizophrenia has gained

wide acceptance and is very useful with regard to prognosis (Phillips, 1953; Kantor and Herron, 1966).

PROCESS schizophrenia which calls to mind the classical descriptions of Langfeldt and Kraepelin, has the following characteristics: (1) Pre-existing *schizoid personality*. A schizoid person is shy, oversensitive, seclusive, and avoids close competitive relations. He may always have been described as eccentric and may daydream a good deal and be unable to express emotions. His social and sexual adjustment is poor. (2) *Insidious onset* which is difficult to date exactly. (3) *No clear precipitating factor* which seems significant enough to have produced psychosis.

In REACTIVE SCHIZOPHRENIA there is: (1) A relatively *acute onset* which is easily dated. The initial symptoms are separated from their time of maximal development by six months or less. (2) *Precipitating factors* that are obviously emotionally charged such as divorce or leaving home. (3) *No pre-existing schizoid personality traits* and therefore a better premorbid social and sexual adjustment than in process schizophrenia. Often there are prominent affective, mainly depressive, symptoms and confusion during the acute episode (Vaillant, 1964; Stephens and Astrup, 1963).

This process-reactive distinction has been validated in many studies (Philips, 1953; Kantor and Herron, 1966), and has been clearly related to prognosis. Reactive schizophrenics have a good prognosis both short-term and long-term; process schizophrenics have a very poor prognosis (Garmezy and Rodnick, 1959; Higgins, 1969; Harrow et al., 1969). It is of interest that the distinguishing criteria are prognostic indicators *only* in schizophrenia, not depression or other nonschizophrenic disorders (Bromet et al., 1971; Rosen et al., 1961).

There is some question about whether the reactive form should be considered schizophrenia. Many of the features that are characteristic of reactive schizophrenia may be encountered in other conditions that can masquerade as schizophrenia. A young psychotic with prominent affective symptoms, for example, may have a primary depression, not schizophrenia. Some of the florid symptoms in such a patient may be related to secondary factors such as sleep deprivation. Features typical of reactive schizophrenia such as the acute onset of confusion and psychosis in a patient with a normal premorbid emotional adjustment have been cited as helpful in ruling out schizophrenia in favor of some other disease process such as subacute encephalitis (Himmelhoch et al., 1970). For these reasons it is conceivable that process schizophrenia may be the real disease and reactive schizophrenia may be something else, perhaps a psychological reaction to stress or an acute encephalopathy. In the absence of a demonstrable biological basis for the diagnosis of schizophrenia this question cannot be resolved; however, the diagnosis of schizophrenia must always be considered tenuous if there has only been a single acute psychotic break. If the disorder becomes chronic, the diagnosis is more certain.

The problem of establishing the relative frequency of occurrence of process and reactive schizophrenia has been very much complicated by variations in the populations studied. In a chronic-state hospital population, there will be a high proportion of "process" schizophrenics. Among schizophrenics admitted for the first time to an acute service, in either a community mental health center or a general hospital, there will be relatively few "process" schizophrenics and more "reactives." For this reason, studies of prognosis in schizophrenia are not necessarily comparable. Many changes in long-term patients attributed to schizophrenia may actually be caused by such aspects of life in a large, poorly staffed state hospital as sensory and emotional deprivation and inadequate nutrition. Thus, while the distinction between process and reactive schizophrenia is probably a valid descriptive one, it should be made at the onset of illness rather than after a patient has been hospitalized for many years because of the possible effects of chronic hospitalization.

COURSE AND NATURAL HISTORY

Kraepelin's original clinical delineation of schizophrenia as a disease entity was made primarily on the basis of its poor prognosis; he postulated that schizophrenic patients manifested a consistently progressive course over time without full recovery. Psychotic patients who recovered were not schizophrenic by definition. In recent years this has been questioned. Manfred Bleuler, for instance, described several patterns of evolution of the disease. One pattern, which varies in severity, is characterized by gradual deterioration over time, and another type is episodic. In the episodic course complete or partial remissions are punctuated by acute exacerbations (Bleuler, 1968).

Bleuler believes that at present the milder chronic conditions have increased in frequency and the severe chronic conditions have diminished. This trend has been observed by others (Grinker, 1972; Remar and Hagopian, 1972), who have also noted shorter psychotic episodes and less bizarre generally more moderate symptoms. While some believe this may be related to the increased use of psychopharmacologic agents, others feel that it represents less repression and greater tolerance of deviance in our contemporary society and take this as evidence that schizophrenia is a culturally determined disorder.

In a study of the charts of schizophrenic patients hospitalized in 1850 and 1950, only minor differences were noted in the symptoms and prognosis (Klaf and Hamilton, 1961). The most marked differences between the two groups were in the kind of delusions the patients had. The patients in 1850 tended to be preoccupied with religion while those of 1950 were more preoccupied with sex. The average age, the proportion of married to single patients, and the incidence of mental illness in the patients' families were the same. Though hospital stays were twice as long in the nineteenth as in the twentieth century, the percentages of cures in both time periods were the same. The remarkable similarity of the symptoms, family history, age of patients, and clinical course lends credence to the disease concept of schizophrenia rather than to a primarily environmental etiology and casts suspicion on the clinical impression that schizophrenia is becoming milder.

While Kraepelin's view that schizophrenia has a uniformly poor outcome is distasteful to those with some therapeutic optimism, the definitive study which proves him wrong has yet to be done. It is notable that Kraepelin studied his patients over a long period of time. Though many of these patients made short-term recoveries they all ultimately deteriorated. Current data suggest that his prognostic view was unnecessarily gloomy for the short term but that it may well be valid for the long-term course. The studies which have examined this point and disagree with Kraepelin suffer from either of two major difficulties: many of the more recent and well-controlled studies are relatively short-term, and the older studies are retrospective and frequently lack accurate diagnostic data.

One of the main obstacles to long-term prospective studies in this country is the strong tradition of divorcing hospital treatment from outpatient treatment. The hospital psychiatrist seldom follows his patient through into outpatient treatment. This is not due to lack of interest but is a logistical problem resulting from the fact that most schizophrenic patients are placed in large state mental hospitals which are far from metropolitan centers. After discharge they return to their homes in the metropolitan areas where outpatient treatment is arranged. This not only complicates patient care but makes good follow-up studies much more difficult.

Table 3-2 is a summary of some of the follow-up studies done over the years. While one would like to think that the introduction of psychopharmacologic agents has greatly affected outcome, and it is clear that improvements have certainly occurred, no "miracles" are as yet evident: In 1963 Peterson studied 177 patients treated with phenothiazines during 1956 to 1958 and showed that over

Table 3-2
Follow-up Studies of Schizophrenic Patients

Author	Dates of Study	Number of Subjects	Results	Length of Follow-up
Bleuler 1950	1898-1905	515	after 1st episode 60% able to support selves (mild deterioration) 22% deteriorated (severe) 18% medium deterioration (medium)	7 years
Freyhan 1955	1920-1955 1940-1955	100 100	54% (sudden onset) out of hospital 24% (gradual onset) out of hospital 71% (sudden onset) out of hospital 49% (gradual onset) out of hospital	35 years 15 years
Israel 1956	1913-1952	4,254	64.1% discharged 24% permanent hospitalization 60% of all discharged never readmitted	40 years
Mandel-brote 1970	1963-1963*	63	46% discharged in 12 months 64% 1st admissions out for 2 years 26% 1st admissions out and discharged but readmitted	3 years
Roder 1970	1951-1955 1956-1960 1951-1952 1959-1960	310	28% of admissions under 5 months' stay 58% of admissions under 5 months' stay 20.8% not readmitted 44.4% not readmitted	3 years

* Phenothiazines introduced in 1954

the next five years one-half of the patients were not readmitted, and for those admitted again another half were not readmitted and so on for each subsequent admission. Twenty-four per cent remained hospitalized at the end of five years (Peterson et al., 1964).

DIFFERENTIAL DIAGNOSIS

Any disease of the central nervous system or disruption of its function (e.g., drugs, sleep deprivation) may have behavioral manifestations. Proper differentiation rests heavily on the type of symptoms present, the mode of onset, the family history of mental illness, the medical history, and the clinical course.

Neurological Diseases

Schizophrenia is not the only condition that can cause disturbances of thinking, though it is by far the most common single cause of such symptoms in young adults. The incidence of schizophrenia in the general population is taken to be approximately one per cent (Srole et al., 1962). Because of this high incidence there is a strong temptation to make the diagnosis of schizophrenia whenever a thought disorder is present. However, schizophrenialike episodes have been described in association with cerebral trauma, tumor, encephalitis, presenile degeneration, other degenerative diseases of gray and white matter, narcolepsy, vascular disorders, and a host of metabolic or toxic disorders such as endocrinopathies, cerebral anoxia, and hypercapnia (Davison and Bagley, 1969). While psychoses are commonly seen with these conditions, they rarely mimic the symptoms of schizophrenia exactly; disorientation, confusion, and fluctuating states of consciousness characteristic of some neurological diseases are seldom encountered in schizophrenia. The difficulty in differentiating schizophrenia from neurologic conditions mainly arises in the initial onset of neurologic illness. Most neurologic illness will either progress to overt neurologic symptoms or else clear completely. So our comments deal mostly with diagnostic problems of acute onset. The mistake often made by inexperienced clinicians is to label as schizophrenic any bizarre, delusional, or mute behavior that cannot be easily explained and is not one of the traditional symptoms associated with a particular medical condition, often overlooking such things as dysmnesia and other signs of neurologic disorder like tremor, myoclonic jerks, and asterixis.

In addition to the presence of disorientation, there are a few simple guidelines for the differentiation of acute neurologic disease from classical schizophrenia. In ACUTE NEUROLOGICAL DISORDERS there is usually: (1) A good premorbid social history. The patient does not have problems at work and his family is generally warm and supportive rather than disturbed, as is so often the case in schizophrenia (Lidz, 1968; Wynne, 1968). (2) An abrupt change in personality, mood, and ability to function at work and at home of less than six months' duration. (3) Rapid fluctuations in mental status. The patient has a clouded sensorium and is disoriented one day, then completely clear the next. While fluctuations can also be seen in some schizophrenics, they are generally not so rapid. Even when the schizophrenic's mental status seems to clear suddenly, he will still show some signs of bizarre behavior or delusional thinking. Although marked fluctuations in mental status are in general more characteristic of acute neurologic disease than schizophrenia, this is not necessarily true of chronic neurologic disease. The fluctuations in mental status of neurological patients may also be accompanied by fluctuating motor behavior. The patient may display aggressive impulses and engage in assaultive behavior at one moment but at the next apologize profusely and try to befriend the people that he has just abused. The mode of behavior during this period frequently has a "driven quality" to it, as has been described in brain-injured patients by Goldstein and Scheerer (1941) and Kahn (1934). (4) A patient with an acute neurological problem is usually unresponsive to psychiatric intervention, whether psychotherapeutic or pharmacologic. Rather than controlling behavior, psychopharmacologic agents may paradoxically precipitate a stuporous or comatose state depending on the underlying condition.

Many patients who present with bizarre behavior and mute states are shunted immediately to the psychiatrist. Even major neurologic signs can be overlooked or interpreted as part of the patient's "functional" disturbance. It goes without saying that marked behavioral aberrations should not blind clinicians to other neurological symptoms.

Drug Reactions

Symptoms suggesting schizophrenia are commonly seen in patients who have taken amphetamines, cocaine, LSD, mescaline, ketamine and belladonna alkaloids. Hallucinations and psychosis may also accompany alcohol and barbiturate withdrawal. These states of intoxication and withdrawal may cause a psychosis without major disorientation (although this is rare) as well as any of the physical changes seen in the neurologically impaired. The presence of visual hallucinations, however, should always suggest the possibility of a drug reaction or a toxic or metabolic encephalopathy. Formed visual hallucinations are unusual in schizophrenia and in diseases which affect the structure of the brain like brain tumors. Auditory hallucinations, on the other hand, are common in schizophrenia and unusual in drug reactions.

Sleep Disorders

Prolonged inability to sleep may produce disorganized thought patterns and even major distortions of reality such as illusions, delusions, and hallucinations. It is possible that this happens only in those with a schizophrenic predisposition. Resumption of a normal sleep pattern in such individuals will resolve their symptoms quickly. Residual thought disorder persists in most schizophrenics even after normal sleep has been restored (Berger and Oswald, 1962; Detre and Jarecki, 1971).

NEUROLOGICAL CHANGES IN SCHIZOPHRENIC PATIENTS

Minor neurologic abnormalities are commonly found in schizophrenia. This is not what one would expect in a "functional" disease and for this reason the presence of such signs is often over-looked or they are considered epiphenomena. One only has to walk through the chronic wards of a large state hospital to be impressed that many of the patients suffer neurologic dysfunction in terms of impaired equilibrium, gait, coordination, and even gross mental retardation. The effects of medication, malnutrition, and multiple electric shocks may have something to do with these abnormalities. Certainly many of the studies of neurologic changes in state hospital populations, where both cause for admission and original symptoms often have been long forgotten, are suspect when they cite a high incidence of neurologic findings in schizophrenics. The few such studies done on acute patients, however, have also documented a significant degree of neurologic dysfunction. Abnormalities include minor motor and sensory ("soft") neurologic signs on physical examination, electroencephalographic abnormalities and "organic" patterns on psychological tests. Heightened "arousal responses" have also been considered by investigators to represent a primary neurological abnormality. MINOR NONLOCALIZING NEUROLOGICAL ABNORMALITIES ("soft signs") have been noted in many studies of acute schizophrenic adult patients (Pollin and Stabenau, 1968; Kennard, 1960; Larsen, 1964; Rochford et al., 1970) and in adolescent schizophrenics (Hertzig and Birch, 1966, 1968).

Rochford examined 65 hospitalized psychiatric patients before any psychotropic medications were administered for the presence of the following minor signs: (1) motor impersistence, (2) stereognosis (3) graphesthesia, (4) extinction during bilateral simultaneous stimulation, (5) bilateral marked hyper-reflexia, (6) coordination defects, (7) disturbance of balance and gait, (8) cortical sensory abnormalities, (9) mild movement disorders, (10) speech defects, (11) abnormal motor activity, (12) defective auditory-visual integration, (13) choreiform movements and adventitious motor overflow (tremor), (14) cranial nerve abnormalities such as slight anisocoria, esotropia, auditory deficit, visual field and retinal defects, and (15) unequivocally abnormal electroencephalograms. He found neurological abnormality in 36.8 per cent of the psychiatric patients (all diagnostic groups). This was significantly different from an age-matched normal control population (5 per cent abnormal signs). Neurologic "soft" signs were found in 65.5 per cent of the schizophrenic patients. By way of comparison, there were no "soft" signs in the patients with primary affective disorders. In 72.5 per cent of the schizophrenics he and his colleagues studied, Pollin found at least one neurologic sign (Pollin and Stabenau, 1968). The most common neurologic abnormalities in Pollin's schizophrenic patients were defects in stereognosis, graphesthesia, difficulty in coordination, balance, and gait, and tremor. There was also some difficulty in the integration of auditory and visual stimuli.

A recent study has confirmed the relationship of minor signs to cognitive defects (Tucker et al., 1973). Fifty-eight consecutive admissions to an acute inpatient psychiatric service were studied with both the Goldstein-Scheerer object sorting test for cognitive disorder and specific sensorimotor portions of the Halstead-Reitan battery (finger agnosia, fingertip writing, tactile form recognition, and the tactile performance test). Forty-three per cent of the entire group of psychiatric patients showed neurologic soft signs. Sixty per cent of those diagnosed as schizophrenic showed neurologic impairment, in contrast to only 21 per cent of the nonschizophrenic psychiatric patients.

Rosenbaum has noted defects in schizophrenic patients with regard to weight discrimination and proprioception. He postulated that these defects are related to "insufficiently articulated proprioceptive signals . . . in schizophrenic persons." The abnormalities he found can be considered "soft signs" similar to those observed in the studies cited above (Rosenbaum, 1971).

Aberrant vestibular function has been widely noted in schizophrenic patients. The vestibular system integrates sensation with motor functions and behavior. Studies made by eleven different groups over the past fifty years have all shown reduced nystagmus in schizophrenic patients in response to caloric and rotational stimulation of the vestibular system (Ornitz, 1970). While the reduced nystagmus response has been related directly to duration of illness in many of the studies, the relationship of vestibular alterations to schizophrenia remains unclear. In some studies (Tice, 1968) auditory and visual hallucinations have followed pharmacological suppression of vestibular sensibility, but direct toxic effects of the drugs elsewhere in the brain were not ruled out in these studies. Prolonged use of psychotropic drugs may induce vestibular changes in chronic patients and this consideration clouds the meaning of the association between vestibular defects and schizophrenia in recent studies. In the older studies, however, the psychotropic drugs were not yet available.

The theory that the behavior of schizophrenics reflects disturbance of the sensory integrative functions of the brain gained support from a series of studies by Silverman (1968) and Buchsbaum and Silverman (1968). These studies show that schizophrenics may actually process incoming stimuli abnormally by attenuating or reducing incoming stimuli. Schizophrenics have a tendency to underestimate tactile, auditory and visual stimuli. While the traditional psychological interpretation of these reduction phenomena has been that they represent a defensive reaction to the schizophrenic's sense of being bombarded by stimuli, the tendency to reduce incoming stimuli may conceivably be a primary defect which produces many of the subjective phenomena common to schizophrenia and sensory deprivation (Vosburg et al., 1959). Silverman postulates that three conditions are associated with and precede such subjective phenomena: (1) either sensory overload or underload, (2) attentiveness to too broad or too narrow range of stimuli (hypo- or hyperattentiveness), and (3) a change in neurophysiologic sensory response systems. Clinical evidence in support of this theory is the observation that acute patients do tend to be in a state of hyperattentiveness to stimuli (McGhie and Chapman,

1961; Chapman, 1966; Tucker et al., 1969; Harrow et al., 1972), as do individuals under the influence of LSD 25. According to Silverman's theory, the cause of schizophrenia is an inability to screen out varied internal and external stimuli. Schizophrenics seem to have a defective sensory filtering mechanism that does not allow them to focus attention on relevant stimuli (Payne, 1960; Callaway, 1970). Inability to focus attention is also one of the features of the altered state of cognitive functioning that occurs during sensory deprivation.

The gross disruptions of perceptual and sensory integrative functions produced by drugs and sensory deprivation regularly lead to psychoticlike states which are at times indistinguishable from schizophrenia. It has long been known that people in isolated situations—arctic camps, solitary prison confinement, patients in iron lungs, and survivors at sea—experience a variety of disturbing subjective alterations. In fact, any environment that is unvarying and offers only limited range of sensory stimuli can give rise to (1) difficulty in focusing and organizing thoughts, (2) illusions and delusions, (3) a sharp sense of the need for variation in extrinsic stimuli, (4) distortion of the sense of time passing, and (5) hallucinatory experiences which are common during prolonged deprivation. These alterations are not limited to the period of deprivation alone but persist briefly after it has ended. Objects continue to appear to swirl, and shapes and lines seem distorted (Solomon et al., 1957). These perceptual experiences associated with sensory deprivation are similar to those described by schizophrenics and by patients with parietal lobe dysfunction.

There is a certain unresolved paradox inherent in this theory of the pathogenesis of schizophrenia. The inability to screen out external stimuli is presented as a primary deficit on the one hand and yet on the other hand it is suggested that alterations in cortical sensory processing produce psychosis by creating a state of sensory deprivation.

EEG

Most of the available data relating electroencephalographic abnormalities to abnormal mental states have been discussed in the section on epilepsy (p. 37). There are no specific EEG changes of either diagnostic or therapeutic use in schizophrenia. A "choppy" EEG (low voltage, 26-50 cps record) in schizophrenic patients has been reported by Davis and Davis (1939), Gibbs et al., (1938) and Hill (1957). The reports of EEG abnormality in schizophrenia range from 5 per cent to 80 per cent with an average of about 25 per cent (Abenson, 1970); however, the vagaries of EEG interpretation and the variability in diagnosing schizophrenia combine to make these figures difficult to interpret. Patients with diagnoses of catatonic schizophrenia seem to show consistently higher rates of EEG abnormality, usually nonspecific slowing (Liberson et al., 1958; Tucker et al., 1965). There have been reports of focal temporal lobe electroencephalographic abnormalities in schizophrenic patients (Hill, 1957; Small et al., 1964; Treffert, 1964; Tucker et al., 1965).

Attempts to study schizophrenics through frequency analysis of the EEG have shown decreased variability and high mean energy content (Goldstein et al., 1963). In several studies this stability or hyperregulation in the EEG's of schizophrenics has been correlated with poor prognosis and dysrhythmic records with a better prognosis (Igert and Lairy, 1962; Yamada, 1960). Many of the EEG studies of schizophrenics are complicated by the treatment given the patients. Fukuda found high voltage slow wave changes after five electroconvulsant treatments (ECT) in 40 to 70 per cent of patients, and in 80 to 87 per cent after 10 ECT's (Fukuda and Matsuda, 1969). While Fukuda reported that almost all EEG's returned to normal in 30 days, Muscovitch disagreed claiming that abnormality lasted at least 10 months (Muscovitch and Katzelenbogen, 1948). The phenothiazines and other psychotropic drugs complicate EEG studies even more; they typically cause slowing of alpha rhythms, increased amplitude with superimposed sharp, fast activity (Steiner and Pollack, 1965). These changes may persist from 10 weeks to three months after medications are stopped (Fink, 1956; Swain and Litteral, 1960). To make interpretation more difficult, usually no predrug EEG's have been recorded. In a study of patients on phenothiazines, Steiner found patterns characteristic of sleep activity in 65 per cent and significant amounts of diffuse delta and theta activity in 43 per cent.

In summary, EEG abnormalities are seen in schizophrenics, especially catatonic schizophrenics, more often than in the general population. This statement seems valid even when allowances are made for the effect of drugs and shock therapy. It is not known whether the schizophrenic process or a presumably underlying biochemical defect causes these electroencephalographic abnormalities. One possibility is that brain damage, which may be reflected in the EEG, could facilitate the development of schizophrenia in individuals who carry a genetic tendency toward the disease.

PSYCHOLOGICAL TESTING FOR SCHIZOPHRENIA

The three types of psychological tests used most frequently in studies of schizophrenia are projective tests (e.g., Rorschach), personality inventories (e.g., MMPI), and performance tests for organicity (e.g., Halstead Organic Test Battery).

PROJECTIVE TESTS present many problems. In the first place they are usually of questionable reliability and validity. Although various standardized scoring techniques have been developed, the information gained differs little from what can be learned in an interview and is in fact no more objective than the clinical impression in determining the presence of a thought disorder (Zubin et al., 1965). Also, it is almost impossible to distinguish neurologic from psychiatric disorders with projective tests. In particular, they fail to reliably separate schizophrenics from neurologic patients (Fisher et al., 1955; Dorken and Kral, 1952). Relying primarily on the verbal responses of patients to vague stimuli, they share the same difficulty in discrimination that the clinical interview has with regard to diagnosis.

PERSONALITY INVENTORIES usually deal with longstanding personality traits. While helpful in raising a suspicion of chronic schizophrenia or schizoid personality, they fail to discriminate acute schizophrenia from acute neurologic syndromes.

PERFORMANCE TESTS for "organicity" do not distinguish the chronic schizophrenic from the neurologically brain-damaged patient. This has been demonstrated quite clearly in two detailed studies using the Halstead Organic Test Battery (Watson et al., 1968) which were unable to distinguish the "organics" from chronic schizophrenics and other studies by Lacks et al. (1970); Vega and Parsons (1970) replicated these findings.

The limited value of psychological tests in differentiating neurological causes of thought disorder from schizophrenia perhaps reflects the "organicity" of the latter disorder.

Arousal

Many studies have identified the schizophrenic as "hyperaroused," a term which refers to an abnormally heightened state of neurophysiological activity. Some feel that this state may actually cause thought disorders. The term "arousal" is not clearly defined but in general refers to a state of alertness with increased physiological measurements of the kind often associated with high levels of anxiety. These include increased galvanic skin resistance, increased muscle tension as measured by electromyography, desynchronization of the EEG with alpha suppression, and increased pulse rate. This evidence of "hyperarousal" has been speculatively linked with statements by acute schizophrenics indicating that they are "flooded" with stimuli, i.e., "When I try to read something, each bit I read starts me thinking in ten different directions at once." It has been suggested that the hyperaroused state leads to a "low threshold for disorganization under increasing stress" (Epstein and Coleman, 1970). The psychophysiological disorganization caused by stimulus overload is hypothesized as the primary causal factor in the thought disturbance typical of schizophrenic patients. When the physiological parameters of "arousal" are studied in samples of schizophrenic and nonschizophrenic patients, however, they correlate more closely with anxiety than with schizophrenia (Tucker et al., 1969). Consequently, "hyperarousal," while frequently present in schizophrenics, is likely to be secondary to anxiety rather than a primary manifestation or cause of schizophrenic thinking.

RELATIONSHIP OF NEUROLOGICAL ABNORMALITIES TO SCHIZOPHRENIA

It is unlikely that the high prevalence of minor neurologic abnormalities in schizophrenic patients is a fortuitous association, for most of the surveys showing a 60 to 70 per cent incidence have been done on large groups of psychiatric patients with different diagnoses, and such minor neurologic findings have been *infrequently* noted in nonschizophrenic patients. The fact that the abnormalities are minor rather than major may explain why they were not reported in the older literature. In our view these signs are minor only in their motor or sensory manifestations; we think that they reflect widespread dysfunction throughout the nervous system and often give rise to serious behavioral and intellectual abnormalities (see p. 126). Not until recent years has it become respectable to consider schizophrenia an organic disease of the brain which might be associated with neurological abnormalities. If this association is not fortuitous there are of course two possibilities: that "minor" brain dysfunction could give rise to schizophrenia or that the schizophrenic process or its treatment could cause the neurologic signs.

The first possibility seems plausible since some neurologic conditions produce symptoms which are characteristic of schizophrenia; the subacute encephalitides and temporal lobe epilepsy, for example, can cause a schizophrenialike psychosis. It could be that such conditions act as precipitating factors in individuals having a specific diathesis for becoming schizophrenic. But this hypothesis is not supported by family studies in cases of the schizophrenialike psychosis of epilepsy or in cases of amphetamine psychosis. If an individual had inherited a schizophrenic tendency, however, he might well be more likely to develop the symptoms of psychosis if he had also sustained brain damage (see p. 90).

While it is possible that neurologic abnormalities in schizophrenics may occasionally represent an organic manifestation of the schizophrenic process or its treatment, in 25 to 30 per cent of schizophrenic patients, medicated and unmedicated, there are no neurologic findings. To resolve the question of the meaning of neurologic abnormalities in schizophrenia it would be necessary to know: (1) Whether the neurologic findings are present over the life time of the patient or become evident at certain developmental stages. (2) Whether these neurologic findings persist during remissions of schizophrenic illness. (3) Whether patients with neurologic abnormalities have a poorer prognosis.

FAMILY STUDIES

The incidence of schizophrenia in the general population is about 1 per cent. The results of epidemiologic surveys of schizophrenia have been very consistent, and all investigators agree that the incidence increases in the families of schizophrenics and is highest in their first-degree relatives. The rate is roughly 10 to 15 per cent in the parents, siblings, and children of schizophrenics. The interpretation of these facts differs, of course. Those who believe that schizophrenia is primarily a functional disorder and who favor an environmental explanation of its development claim that the higher incidence in relatives can be credited to the exposure of children to the abnormal environment created by sick adults. Those favoring a genetic hypothesis believe that these figures reflect a genetic influence. Most psychiatrists in this country take the middle view that schizophrenia is a functional illness influenced by genetic factors.

Many studies of families of schizophrenics have been done. Virtually all agree that approximately half of the parents of schizophrenics display serious personality disorders. Lidz (1968) found that 60 per cent of the patients' parents displayed "psychotic traits." Alanen (1968) reported that 63 per cent of the mothers of schizophrenics were "more seriously ill than psychoneurotic." These authors favor an environmental hypothesis of the etiology of schizophrenia, but their data could serve equally well to support a genetic hypothesis.

A major criticism of the view that schizophrenia is a functional disorder is that many schizophrenics do not come from an abnormal environment. In our opinion, an even stronger objection to the view that psychogenic stress or life experience can cause schizophrenia is that no *specific* environmental circumstances have been identified to which an increased morbidity risk of schizophrenia can be attributed. Many psychogenic theories have been proposed over the last 50 years but no predictions of psychogenic risk factors have ever been made or verified. Most studies which purport to show the effect of environment on the development of schizophrenia do not include adequate control groups and do not distinguish the effect of a schizophrenic child on his parents' mental state from the effect of the parents on the child.

A few jots of evidence do exist which have been interpreted as suggesting an important role for the psychological environment in the causation of schizophrenia. Hollingshead and Redlich (1954) have shown that prevalence rates for schizophrenia are eight times higher in lower classes (Class V) than in the highest class (I). This, it has been said, implies that the lower class environment contains unfavorable factors which are etiologically important. It has not proved possible to substantiate this interpretation of the data of Hollingshead and Redlich. A study of a national (British) sample of schizophrenics (Goldberg and Morrison, 1963), which confirmed the higher prevalence of the disease in the lower classes, found that the patients' fathers had had an occupational distribution corresponding to the general population. In other words, the low social class of the patients is likely to be the result of a downward dirft occurring during the premorbid phase or the insidious early stages of illness. There is abundant evidence that such a prepsychotic drift occurs (Slater and Cowie, 1971; Pollack et al., 1966; Bower et al., 1960; and Prout and White, 1956).

Another bit of evidence which has been interpreted as supporting the environmental hypothesis is the finding that schizophrenia is more common amongst the mothers of schizophrenic offspring than amongst their fathers. This, along with descriptive studies by Alanen (1958) and others which indicate a high rate of nonschizophrenic psychiatric disturbance in the mothers of schizophrenics has been a main pillar of support for the "schizophrenic mother" variant of the environmental hypothesis. According to this theory, the patient's mother causes schizophrenia by the harmful way she relates to her child. However, there are alternative explanations for the data on which this theory is based. The higher incidence of schizophrenia in mothers of schizophrenics may reflect the facts that reproductive capacity is adversely affected by schizophrenia but women marry at an earlier age than men and tend to become schizophrenic at a later age than men. These factors increase the interval between the age of marriage and onset of psychosis in women as compared to men. Since the requirement for an active role in reproduction is greater in men than women, schizophrenic women would be more likely to produce children than schizophrenic men, even after psychosis had developed. Very much against the "schizophrenic mother hypothesis" is the evidence that the children of schizophrenic fathers run the same risk of developing the disease as the children of schizophrenic mothers (Slater and Cowie, 1971).

Twin studies have added to the evidence against the environmental hypothesis and support the genetic. There have been 11 major twin studies of schizophrenia. These studies were done in the U.S., the United Kingdom, Japan, Germany, and Scandinavia. In all but one (Tienari, 1963) the incidence of schizophrenia is much higher in monozygotic than dizygotic twins of schizophrenics (Gottesman and Shields, 1966). The overall incidence of schizophrenia in the monozygotic twins of schizophrenics is 61 per cent. This represents 249 concordant twins out of 409 twin pairs. In the dizygotic twins studied there was a 12 per cent concordance rate (70 out of 571 pairs). In other words, the incidence of schizophrenia in dizygotic twins is the same as in nontwin siblings of schizophrenics. The unique prospective study of Gottesman and Shields, a particularly careful one, was based on consecutive admissions to outpatient and short-stay inpatient facilities over a 16-year period and thus included mild and severe cases. By adhering to strict criteria of monozygoticity and spelling out in detail the criteria on which they based their assessment of the severity of the disease, this study met the major criticisms of earlier twin research in schizophrenia. It indicated a 42 per cent incidence in the monozygotic twins of schizophrenics and a 9 per cent incidence in dizygotic twins. However, monozygotic concordance for severe schizophrenia was 77 per cent contrasted to 27 per cent for mild schizophrenia. The corresponding figures for the dizygotic probands were 15 per cent and 10 per cent.

The obvious interpretation of these facts is that schizophrenia is a genetic illness but objections to this interpretation have been raised to this effect: since parents tend to treat monozygotic twins in an identical manner and to treat dizygotic twins differently, the harmful influence (unnamed) which derives from the psychic environment is likely to affect monozygotics in the same way but will be unequally felt by dizygotes. This hypothesis can be tested by studies of monozygotic twins (one of whom has become schizophrenic), separated in the first year of life and raised apart. Slater and Cowie (1971) reviewed all reports of such cases and found that of 12 monozygotic pairs, 9 were concordant. While these numbers are small, the high concordance rate argues strongly against a significant psychoenvironmental influence in schizophrenia.

Another approach to testing the environmental hypothesis was taken in a study of the psychosocial adjustment of 47 adults who had been born to schizophrenic mothers and permanently separated from their mothers during the first days of life (Heston, 1966). They were compared to 50 control adults with nonschizophrenic mothers who had also been permanently separated from their natural mothers in the first few days of life. The comparison was based on a review of school, police, army, and hospital records, plus a personal interview and personality testing (MMPI). I.Q. testing and social-class determination were also done and three psychiatrists independently rated the subjects. In this study schizophrenia was significantly more prevalent in the individuals born to schizophrenic mothers. Five out of 47 persons with schizophrenic mothers were schizophrenic. No cases of schizophrenia were found in the 50 control subjects. The age-corrected rate for schizophrenia in the experimental group was 16.6 per cent, a finding consistent with that of all family studies which have been done on children raised by their schizophrenic biological parents. In addition, serious psychosocial disability, that is, psychiatric diagnosis other than schizophrenia, was found in approximately one-half of the persons born to schizophrenic mothers. Many had been discharged from the armed forces for behavioral reasons; others had police records or alcoholism. The diagnosis of sociopathic personality was made more than four times as often in the experimental group, in which five times as many persons spent more than one year in a penal or psychiatric institution.

These findings have been substantiated independently by a similar study (Rosenthal et al., 1968). In this study many more schizophrenics were discovered in a group of adopted individuals one of whose biologic parents was schizophrenic than in a matched control group of adopted persons neither of whose parents had the disease. A parallel study that compared the incidence and type of psychopathology in adoptive parents of schizophrenics, biological parents of schizophrenics and controls clearly demonstrated a qualitative and quantitative increase in the severity of psychopathology among biological as opposed to adoptive parents of schizophrenics (Wender et al., 1968).

These studies do more than merely offer support for a theory about genetic influence in schizophrenia. They indicate that it is a genetic disease. They offer no support for the view that psychosocial environment plays any role in determining the risk of developing schizophrenia in individuals who are genetically at high risk. The child of a schizophrenic has the same chance of developing the disease whether he is raised by his schizophrenic parent or in a normal environment.

Those who believe in the importance of environmental influences in the development of schizophrenia have claimed that the failure of concordance rates for monozygotic twins to reach 100 per cent is evidence in favor of their position. For if schizophrenia were a genetic disease uninfluenced by the emotional environment concordance should be 100 per cent in monozygotic pairs. This criticism of the genetic view is not valid as experience with epilepsy has shown. The genetic tendency to petit mal and other forms of epilepsy demonstrated by EEG studies is transmitted as an autosomal dominant trait. Yet concordance rates for clinical epilepsy in monozygotic pairs do not reach one hundred per cent. No one can claim that emotional factors can explain this discrepancy in concordance rates for epilepsy but acquired brain damage in one sibling often seems to be responsible. Using this analogy and the well-established fact that multiple pregnancies result in a higher incidence of neurologic complications, one can hypothesize that acquired brain damage in an individual with a genetic tendency for schizophrenia might allow full expression of the gene in that individual. If this were so, the incidence of low birth weight and factors known to be associated with brain damage would presumably be higher in the schizophrenic twin of a discordant monozygotic pair (Campion and Tucker, 1973).

This expectation has been realized in a study of 15 such pairs by Pollin and Stabenau (1968). In eleven of the 15 schizophrenics there were lower birth weights than found in their monozygotic twin as well as disordered early feeding and sleep patterns. Two of the remaining four suffered severe early childhood illnesses (prolonged cyanosis caused by an exposure to gas in one and Rocky Mountain Spotted Fever in the other). There was a marked preponderance of minor neurological abnormalities in the schizophrenic twins.

Thus, there would certainly appear to be an environmental influence in schizophrenia if by "environmental" one means acquired brain damage rather than psychosocial factors such as emotional deprivation.

The idea that brain damage might allow full expression of a gene for schizophrenia can be invoked to explain the high incidence of neurologic and electroencephalographic abnormalities seen in schizophrenic patients. Available data suggest that there might be an autosomal dominant gene for schizophrenia, as there is for petit mal epilepsy, whose penetrance varies with the age of the individual and whose expressivity is in large part determined by the presence of acquired brain damage and by other genes which influence personality, adaptability, and other brain functions. The difference between this view and the "polygenic" theory of the inheritance of schizophrenia is minimal. According to the polygenic model a variety of genes and acquired traits determine an individual's liability to the disease. If an individual inherits many "bad" genes, he is likely to have severe schizophrenia. A milder schizophrenic condition would result if fewer of the offending agents were present and, in the most mild cases resulting from a small number of such factors a variety of nonschizophrenic alterations in behavior or personality could develop. The relative merits of the polygenic and single gene hypotheses have been discussed extensively by Slater and Cowie (1971).

EFFECT OF EMOTIONAL FACTORS UPON SCHIZOPHRENIA

Psychosocial factors can affect schizophrenics, as they may affect diabetics or epileptics, by augmenting illness, coloring the content of the symptoms, and by increasing the frequency and severity of the symptoms. Psychosocial factors can undoubtedly be helpful in terms of treatment or supportive environment, just as they can be harmful.

As Cannon pointed out long ago, emotional factors may cause physiological changes (Cannon, 1915). Acute stress reactions may be associated with hormonal changes and increases in blood pressure, pulse rate, and respiratory rate. The clinical impression that anxiety may precipitate seizures in epileptics seems well substantiated, though the mechanism by which anxiety influences the frequency and severity of seizures are only partly understood. There may be a "limbic reflex" in which excitatory impulses alter the resting potentials of neurons in critical regions—lowering thresholds and producing uncontrolled discharge. On the other hand, it is known that anxiety-induced hyperventilation can precipitate seizures by causing either respiratory alkalosis or cerebral anoxia secondary to decreased cerebral blood flow.

The clinical impression of psychiatrists that life stresses are associated with decompensation in patients with a pre-existing schizophrenic diathesis also seems fairly well substantiated, though it must be remembered that all such clinical impressions are scientifically suspect and involve "post hoc" reasoning. While the basis for this remains obscure, it may relate to a possible alteration of bio-genic amines in critical areas of the hypothalamus and the reticular activating and limbic systems. Many examples could be given of schizophrenia and indeed of other psychoses in which environmental stresses may have determined the timing, severity, and content of the symptomatology. However, it is quite another thing to go on to claim, as many do, that emotional factors cause the psychotic condition.

TREATMENT

Aside from the environmental and psychotherapeutic aspects of management, it is unquestionable that the use of the major antipsychotic drugs (phenothiazines, thioxanthene, butylphenuones, and reserpine) is essential to the treatment of acute schizophrenics. Not only are these drugs more effective than placebos for schizophrenics (Klein and Davis, 1969), but they are also more effective than any type of psychotherapy alone (May, 1968; Grinspoon et al., 1968). In acute schizophrenia or chronic schizophrenia with an acute exacerbation, the response to the phenothiazines is so prompt and consistent that the diagnosis is likely to be incorrect if there is not a favorable response to treatment. However, in process schizophrenia—chronic and undifferentiated, simple and hebephrenic schizophrenias—there is usually no significant response to treatment.

While there are many major tranquilizers, controlled studies show little difference in their effectiveness. The clinician should probably acquaint himself with one or two of these drugs (preferably one of the phenothiazines that is marketed in pill, elixir, and injectable form) so as to become familiar with the effects, onset of action and side effects. Perhaps the most common error in the use of phenothiazines is not using a large enough dose.

While the exact site of action of the major tranquilizers is unclear, the behavioral effects are slowly being defined. In a large

Schizophrenia 93

fective in controlling were associative deficits such as overinclusive thinking and poor abstracting ability. Also, withdrawal, autism and such symptoms as hallucinations, hostility, and uncooperativeness respond well to major tranquilizers. The drugs were not as effective for such symptoms as blunted affect, paranoid ideas, or grandiosity, which nevertheless can sometimes be moderated with phenothiazines (Chapman and Knowles, 1964; Goldberg et al., 1965; Saretsky, 1966; Shimkunas et al., 1966).

study sponsored by the NIMH, the symptoms these drugs were ef-

REFERENCES

Abenson, M. H. EEG's in chronic schizophrenia. Brit. J. Psychiat. 116: 421-25, 1970.

Alanen, Y. O. The mothers of schizophrenic patients. Acta Psychiat. Scand. Suppl. 124, 1958.

———. From the mothers of schizophrenic patients to interactional family dynamics. In: David Rosenthal and Seymour Kety, eds., The Transmission of Schizophrenia. Pergamon Press, London, 1968.

American Psychiatric Association. Diagnostic and Statistical Manual of Mental Disorders. Second ed., American Psychiatric Association, Washington, D.C., 1968.

Arieti, S. Interpretation of Schizophrenia. Brunner, New York, 1955.

Beck, A. T., C. H. Ward, M. Mandelson, J. E. Mock, and J. K. Erbaugh. Reliability of psychiatric diagnosis: 2. A study of consistency of clinical judgments and ratings. Amer. J. Psychiat. 119: 351-57, 1962.

Berger, R. J. and I. Oswald. Effects of sleep deprivation, subsequent sleep and dreaming. Brit. J. Psychiat. 108: 457-65, 1962.

Bleuler, E. Dementia Praecox or the Group of Schizophrenias. Zinkin (trans.). International Universities Press, New York, 1950.

Bleuler, M. A 23 Year Longitudinal Study of 208 Schizophrenics. In: D. Rosenthal and S. Kety, eds., Transmission of Schizophrenia. Pergamon Press, London, pp. 3-14, 1968.

Bower, E. M., T. A. Shellhamer, J. M. Daily. School characteristics of male adolescents who later become schizophrenics. Amer. J. Orthopsychiat. 30: 712-29, 1960.

Bromet, E., M. Harrow, G. J. Tucker. Factors related to short-term prognosis in schizophrenia and depression. Arch. Gen. Psychiat. 25: 148-54, 1971.

Buchsbaum, M. and J. Silverman. Stimulus intensity control and cortical evoked response. Psychosom. Med. 30: 12-22, 1968.

Callaway, E. Schizophrenia and interference. Arch. Gen. Psychiat. 22: 193-208, 1970.

Cameron, N. Personality Development and Psychopathology. Houghton Mifflin Co., Boston, 1963.

Campion, E. W. and G. J. Tucker. A note on twin studies, schizophrenia and neurological impairment. Arch. Gen. Psychiat. 35: 60-65, 1973.

Cannon, W. B. Bodily Changes in Pain, Hunger, Fear and Rage. Appleton-Century-Crofts, New York, 1915.

Chapman, L. J. and R. R. Knowles. The effects of phenothiazine on disordered thought in schizophrenia. J. Consult. Psychol. 28(2): 165-69, 1964.

Chapman, J. The early symptoms of schizophrenia. Brit. J. Psychiat. 112: 225-51, 1966.

Davis, P. A. and H. Davis. Electroencephalograms of psychotic patients. Am. J. Psychiat. 95: 1007, 1939.

Davison, K. and C. R. Bagley. Schizophrenia-like Psychoses Associated with Organic Disorders of the Central Nervous System: A Review of the Literature. In: R. N. Herrington, ed., Current Problems in Neuropsychiatry. Brit. J. Psychiat., Special Pub. No. 4. Ashford, Kent, Headley Bros., 1969.

Detre, T. and H. Jarecki. Modern Psychiatric Treatment. J. B. Lippincott, New York, 1971.

Dörken, H. and V. A. Kral. The psychological differentiation of organic brain lesions and their localization by means of the Rorschach Test. Am. J. Psychiat. 108: 764-70, 1952.

Epstein, S. and M. Coleman. Drive theories of schizophrenia. Psychosom. Med. 32: 113-40, 1970.

Feighner, J. P., E. Robins, S. B. Guze, R. A. Woodruff, G. Winokur, and R. Munoz. Diagnostic criteria for use in psychiatric research. Arch. Gen. Psychiat. 26: 57-63, 1972.

Fink, M. and R. C. Kahn. Relation of EEG delta activity to behavioral response in electroshock. Arch. Neurol. Psychiat. 78: 516-25, 1956.

Fisher, J., T. A. Gonda, and K. Little. The Rorschach and central nervous system pathology. Am. J. Psychiat. 111: 487-92, 1955.

Freyhan, F. A. Course and outcome of schizophrenia. Amer. J. Psychiat. 111: 161-69, 1955.

Fukuda, T. and Y. Matsuda. Comparative characteristics of slow wave EEG, autonomic function and clinical picture in typical and atypical schizophrenia during and following electroconvulsive treatment. Int. Pharmacopsychiat. 3: 13-41, 1969.

Garmezy, N. and E. H. Rodnick. Premorbid adjustment and performance in schizophrenia: Implications for interpreting heterogeneity in schizophrenia. J. Nerv. Ment. Dis. 129: 450-66, 1959.

Gibbs, F. A., E. L. Gibbs, and W. G. Lennox. Likeness of cortical-dysrhythmias of schizophrenia and psychomotor epilepsy. Am. J. Psychiat. 95: 255, 1938.

Goldberg, E. M. and S. L. Morrison. Schizophrenia and social class. Brit. J. Psychiat. 109: 785-802, 1963.

Goldberg, S. C., G. Klerman, and J. Cole. Changes in schizophrenic psychopathology and ward behavior as a function of phenothiazine treatment. Brit. J. Psychiat., 111: 120-33, 1965.

Goldstein, K. and M. Scheerer. Abstract and concrete behavior, an experimental study with special tests. Psychological Monographs, 53 (2, Whole No. 239), 1941.

————. Methodological Approach to the Study of Schizophrenic Thought Disorder. In: J. S. Kasanin, ed., Language and Thought In Schizophrenia. W. W. Norton & Co., New York, 1944.

————. Concerning the concreteness in schizophrenia. J. Abnormal & Soc. Psychol. 57: 146-48, 1958.

Goldstein, L., H. B. Murphree, A. A. Sugerman, C. C. Pfeiffer, E. H. Jenney. Quantitative electroencephalographic analysis of naturally occurring (schizophrenic) and drug-induced psychotic states in human males. Clin. Pharmacol. & Therapeutics 4(1): 10-21, 1963.

Gottesman, I. I. and J. Shields. Schizophrenia in twins: 16 years consecutive admissions to a psychiatric clinic. Brit. J. Psychiat. 112: 809-18, 1966.

Grinker, R. R. Changing Styles in Psychiatric Syndromes: Psychoses and Borderline States. Presented at 125th Annual Meeting, American Psychiatric Association, Dallas, Texas, May 1972.

Grinspoon, L., J. R. Ewalt, and R. Shader. Psychotherapy and pharmacotherapy in chronic schizophrenia. Am. J. Psychiat. 124: 1645-52, 1968.

Harrow, M., G. J. Tucker, and E. Bromet. Short-term prognosis of schizophrenic patients. Arch. Gen. Psychiat. 21: 195-202, 1969.

————, ————, and D. Adler. Concrete and idiosyncratic thinking in acute schizophrenic patients. Arch. Gen. Psychiat. 26: 433-39, 1972.

————, G. J. Tucker, and P. Shield. Stimulus overinclusion in schizophrenic disorders. Arch. Gen. Psychiat. 27: 40-45, 1972.

Hertzig, M. A. and H. G. Birch. Neurologic organization in psychiatrically disturbed adolescent girls. Arch. Gen. Psychiat. 15: 590-99, 1966.

—— and ——. Neurologic organization in psychiatrically disturbed adolescents. Arch. Gen. Psychiat. 19: 528-37, 1968.

Heston, L. L. Psychiatric disorders in foster home reared children of schizophrenic mothers. Brit. J. Psychiat. 112: 819-25, 1966.

Higgins, J. Process-reactive schizophrenia recent developments. J. Nerv. Ment. Dis. 149: 450-72, 1969.

Hill, D. Electroencephalogram in Schizophrenia. In: D. Richter, ed., Schizophrenia: Somatic Aspects. Pergamon Press, London, 1957.

Hollingshead, A. B. and F. C. Redlich. Social stratification and schizophrenia. Am. Sociol. Rev. 19: 302-6, 1954.

Hordern, A., M. G. Sandifer, L. M. Green, and G. C. Tinbury. Psychiatric diagnosis: British and North American concordance on stereotypes of mental illness. Brit. J. Psychiat. 114: 935-44, 1968.

Igert, C. and G. C. Lairy. Intêret prognostique de l'EEG au cours de l'évolutions des schizophrènes. Electroencephlog. & Clin. Neurophysiol. 14: 183-90, 1962.

Israel, R. H. and N. A. Johnson. Discharge and readmission rates in 4,254 consecutive first admissions of schizophrenia. Am. J. Psychiat. 112: 903-9, 1956.

Kahn, E. Organic driveness; a brainstem syndrome and an experience with case reports. New Eng. J. Med. 210: 748-56, 1934.

Kantor, R. E. and W. G. Herron. Reactive and Process Schizophrenia. Science and Behavior Books, Palo Alto, Cal., 1966.

Kennard, M. Value of equivocal signs in neurological diagnosis. Neurology 10: 753-64, 1960.

Klaf, F. S. and J. G. Hamilton. Schizophrenia—a hundred years ago and today. J. Ment. Science 107: 819-27, 1961.

Klein, D. F. and J. M. Davis. Diagnosis and Drug Treatment of Psychiatric Disorders. Williams & Wilkins Co. Baltimore, 1969.

Kraepelin, E. Dementia Praecox and Paraphrenia. 8th German ed. Livingstone, Edinburgh, 1925.

Lacks, P. B., J. Colbert, M. Harrow, and J. Levine. Further evidence concerning the diagnostic accuracy of the Halstead Organic Test Battery. J. Clin. Psychol. 26: 480-81, 1970.

Larsen, V. Physical characteristics of disturbed adolescents. Arch. Gen. Psychiat. 10: 55-64, 1964.

Liberson, W. T., I. W. Scherer, and C. J. Klett. Further observations on EEG effects of chlorpromazine. Electroenceph. Clin. Neurophysiol. 10: 192-93, 1958.

Lidz, T. The Family, Language, and the Transmission of Schizophrenia. In: D. Rosenthal and S. Kety, eds., Transmission of Schizophrenia. Pergamon Press, London, 1968.

McGhie, A. and J. Chapman. Disorders of attention and perception in early schizophrenia. Brit. Med. Psychol. 34: 103-16, 1961.

Mandelbrote, B. M. and K. L. K. Trick. Social and clinical factors in the outcome of schizophrenia. Acta Psychiat. Scand., 46: 24-34, 1970.

May, P. R. A. Treatment of Schizophrenia. Science House, New York, 1968.

Mayer-Gross, W., E. Slater, and M. Roth. Clinical Psychiatry. Williams & Wilkins Co., Baltimore, 3rd ed., 1969.

Muscovitch A. and T. Katzelenbogen. Electroshock therapy, clinical and EEG studies. J. Nerv. Ment. Dis., 107: 517, 1948.

Ornitz, E. Vestibular dysfunction in schizophrenia and childhood autism. Comprehensive Psychiat. 11: 159-73, 1970.

Payne, R. W. Cognitive Abnormalities. In: H. J. Eysenck, ed., Handbook of Abnormal Psychology. Pitman, London, 1960.

Peterson, D. B., M. O. Fulton, and G. W. Olson. First admitted schizophrenics in drug era. Arch. Gen. Psychiat. 11: 137-44, 1964.

Phillips, L. Case history data and prognosis in schizophrenia. J. Nerv. Ment. Dis. 117: 515-25, 1953.

Pollack, M., M. G. Woerner, W. Goodman, and I. M. Greenberg. Childhood development patterns of hospitalized adult schizophrenic and nonschizophrenic patients and their siblings. Am. J. Orthopsychiat. 36: 510-17, 1966.

Pollin, W. and J. Stabenau. Biological, Psychological, and Historical Differences in a Series of Monozygotic Twins Discordant for Schizophrenia. In: D. Rosenthal and S. Kety, eds., Transmission of Schizophrenia. Pergamon Press, London, 1968.

Prout, C. T. and M. A. White. The schizophrenic's sibling. J. Nerv. Ment. Dis. 123: 162-70, 1956.

Remar, E. M. and P. B. Hagopian. Changing Clinical Syndromes: Forty-Year Perspective. Presented at 125th Annual Meeting of American Psychiatric Association, Dallas, Texas, May 1972.

Rochford, J. M., T. Detre, G. J. Tucker, and M. Harrow. Neuropsychological impairments in functional psychiatric diseases. Arch. Gen. Psychiat. 22: 114-19, 1970.

Roder, E. A prognostic investigation of female schizophrenic patients discharged from Sct. Hans Hospital, Dept. D, during the decade 1951-1960. Acta Psychiat. Scand. 46: 50-63, 1970.

Rosen, B., D. F. Klein, S. Levenstein, and S. P. Shahinian. Social competence and posthospital outcome among schizophrenic and nonschizophrenic psychiatric patients. J. Abnormal Psychol. 74: 401-4, 1969.

Rosenbaum, G. Feedback Mechanisms in Schizophrenia. In: Lafayette Clinic Studies on Schizophrenia. Wayne State University Press, Detroit, 1971, pp. 163-85.

Rosenthal, D., P. H. Wender, S. Kety, F. Schulsinger, J. Welner and L. Østergaard. Schizophrenics' Offspring Reared in Adoptive Homes. In: D. Rosenthal and S. Kety, eds., Transmission of Schizophrenia. Pergamon Press, London, 1968.

Sanua, V. D. Sociocultural Aspects. In L. Bellak and L. Loeb, eds., The Schizophrenic Syndrome. Grune and Stratton, New York, 1969, pp. 256-310.

Saretsky, T. Effects of chlorpromazine on primary-process thought manifestations. J. Abnormal Psychol. 71(4): 247-52, 1966.

Schneider, K. Clinical Psychopathology. M. W. Hamilton (trans.). Grune and Stratton, New York, 1959.

Shimkunas, A. M., M. D. Gyntherm, and K. Smith. Abstracting ability of schizophrenics before and during phenothiazine therapy. Arch. Gen. Psychiat. 14: 79-83, 1966.

Silverman, J. A paradigm for the study of altered states of consciousness. Brit. J. Psychiat. 114: 1201-18, 1968.

Slater, E. and V. Cowie. The Genetics of Mental Disorders. Oxford University Press, London, 1971.

Small, J. G., I. F. Small, and W. R. P. Surphils. Temporal EEG abnormalities in acute schizophrenia. Am. J. Psychiat. 121: 262, 1964.

Solomon, P., P. H. Leiderman, J. Mendelson, and D. Wexler. Sensory deprivation: a review. Am. J. Psychiat. 114: 357-63, 1957.

Srole, L., et al. Mental Health in the Metropolis. McGraw-Hill Book Co., New York, 1962.

Steiner, W. G. and S. L. Pollack. Limited usefulness of EEG as a diagnostic aid in psychiatric cases receiving tranquilizing drug therapy. Progress in Brain Research, 16: 97-105, 1965. Amsterdam, Elsevier Publishing Co.

Stephens, J. H. and C. Astrup. Prognosis in "process" and "nonprocess" schizophrenia. Am. J. Psychiat. 119: 945-52, 1963.

Sullivan, H. S. Conceptions of Modern Psychiatry. W. W. Norton & Co., New York, 1953.

Swain, J. M. and E. B. Litteral. Prolonged effect of chlorpromazine:

EEG findings in a senile group. J. Nerv. Ment. Dis., 131: 550-53, 1960.

Tice, L. F.   New drugs of 1967. Am. J. Pharm., 140: 4-21, 1968.

Tienari, P.   Psychiatric illness in identical twins. Acta Psychiat. Scand. Suppl. 171, 1963.

Treffert, D. A.   Psychiatric patient with EEG temporal lobe focus. Am. J. Psychiat. 120: 765-71, 1964.

Tucker, G. J., T. Detre, M. Harrow and G. H. Glaser.   Behavior and symptoms of psychiatric patients and the electroencephalogram. Arch. Gen. Psychiat., 12: 278-86, 1965.

———, M. Harrow, T. Detre, and B. Hoffman.   Perceptual experiences in schizophrenic and nonschizophrenic patients. Arch. Gen. Psychiat. 20: 159-66, 1969.

———, and E. W. Campion, P. A. Kelleher, and P. M. Silberfarb. The Relationship of Subtle Neurologic Impairments to Disturbances of Thinking. Presented at the 2nd Congress of the International College of Psychosomatic Medicine, Amsterdam, June 1973.

Vaillant, G. E.   Prospective prediction of schizophrenic remission. Arch. Gen. Psychiat. 11: 509-18, 1964.

Vega, A. and O. A. Parsons.   Cross-validation of the Halstead-Reitan tests for brain damage. J. Consult. Psychol. 31: 619-25, 1967.

Von Domarus, E.   The Specific Laws of Logic in Schizophrenia. In J. S. Kasamin, ed., Language and Thought in Schizophrenia: Collected Papers. University of California Press, Berkeley, 1944.

Vosburg, R., N. Fraser, and J. Guehl.   Sensory deprivation and image formation. Psychiat. Commun. 4: 157-70, 1959.

Vygotsky, L. S.   Thought and Language. E. Hanfman, and G. Vakar, eds. and trans. John Wiley & Sons, New York, 1962.

Watson, C. G., R. W. Thomas, D. Andersen, and J. Felling.   Differentiation of organics from schizophrenics at two chronicity levels by use of the Reitan-Halstead Organic Test Battery. J. Consult. & Clin. Psychol. 32(6): 679-84, 1968.

Wender, P. H., D. Rosenthal, and S. Kety.   A Psychiatric Assessment of the Adoptive Parents of Schizophrenics. In: D. Rosenthal and S. Kety, eds., Transmission of Schizophrenia. Pergamon Press, London, 1968.

Wynne, L. C.   Methodologic and Conceptual Issues in the Study of Schizophrenics and Their Families. In: D. Rosenthal and S. Kety, eds., Transmission of Schizophrenia. Pergamon Press, London, 1968.

Yamada, T.   Heterogeneity of schizophrenia as demonstrable in EEG. Bull. Osaka Med. Sch., 6: 107-46, 1960.

Zubin, J., L. D. Eron, and F. Schumer.   An Experimental Approach to Projective Techniques. John Wiley & Sons, New York, 1965.

Chapter 4

ORGANIC BRAIN SYNDROMES

The terms *organic brain syndrome* and *dementia* are applied to those acquired disorders of thinking and other cognitive functions that are believed to arise from altered structure or function of the nervous system and thus stand opposed to the "functional" disorders. The inadequacy of this distinction is immediately apparent: all "functional" disorders must be the result of disordered brain activity. In conventional usage "organic brain syndrome" and "dementia" refer to disorders of mentation caused by diseases traditionally considered to lie within the province of neurologists, and it is in this sense that we will use the term in this chapter. The symptoms of dementia can be similar to those of amentia or congenital mental retardation, but the first term implies the loss of previously acquired mental abilities and hence has different diagnostic and therapeutic implications.

Neurologic diseases that may cause dementia characteristically impair orientation and memory when dysfunction is extensive, but when it is less serious, more subtle changes of personality and intellectual functioning may precede disorientation and dysmnesia. While disturbances of orientation to time, place, person, and of memory are perhaps the hallmarks of organic brain syndromes, it is important to note that other types of dysfunction are also characteristic. Impairment of verbal, spatial, and numerical abilities may become manifest in disturbances of language function, of calculation, and of the ability to orient oneself or objects in space. Impairment may also be evident in personality and in the level of consciousness or "vigilance," at which a patient seems to be functioning. Thus, the diagnosis of an organic brain syndrome involves an evaluation of: (1) perception, (2) memory, (3) orientation, (4) verbal, spatial, and numerical ability (5) level of consciousness and (6) change in personality. It is important to note that disturbances of these functions may involve only one or all areas and when more than one is involved, the degree of dysfunction in each may vary in severity.

FACTORS IN CONTENT

Three major factors determine the manifestations of an organic brain syndrome: *the amount of tissue destroyed, the location of the lesion in the brain,* and *the nature of the disease process.* There has been a classical argument in neurology as to whether location or amount of damage is the more important factor. On one side have been those who equated structure with function and attempted to identify "centers" or anatomical loci of particular functions in the brain. On the other side stand those who agree with Lashley (1929) that all cortical regions of the brain are equipotential for intelligence and that the mass of brain tissue destroyed is therefore much more important than the location of the lesion. On the basis of evidence which will be presented below, it is clear that anatomical specialization to some degree does exist in the human brain but is not sufficient to provide functional divisions for many intellectual abilities.

Amount of Destruction

Chapman and Wolff (1959) made the most extensive, systematic test of Lashley's hypothesis in human beings. Their classic study correlated measured brain tissue removal during surgery for tumors with postoperative intellectual deficiency. When brain damage was not extensive, involving less than 120g of cortical tissue, adaptive capacities were found to be impaired even though orientation and memory remained intact. Chapman and Wolff divided the symptoms of such "minimal" brain damage into four categories: (1) *expression of needs, appetites, and drives:* There is less seeking of challenges and adventure, less imagination, less desire for human associations and sexual activity, along with a passive acceptance of circumstances and a lack of aspirations in brain-damaged patients. When mild, such symptoms mimic depression and, indeed patients with slight brain damage often are depressed; the depression may be a reaction to or a manifestation of their deficit. When brain damage is severe, inability to express needs may even extend to such basic needs as food, shelter, and warmth. (2) *Capacity to adapt for the achievement of goals:* Brain-damaged individuals have a decreased ability to anticipate either dangerous or propitious circumstances, to plan, arrange, invent, postpone, modulate, or discriminate in achieving goals. Business failure or unwise sexual liaisons, for example, may occur in the course of advancing disease and may cause great distress to the patient's family, especially when he seems normal in other ways. (3) *Integration of socially appropriate reactions of defense under stress* and (4) *Capacity to recover promptly from the effects of stress.* Deficits in the third and fourth categories can lead to the catastrophic reaction first noted in war veterans who had apparently recovered from brain injuries. When confronted with an arithmetic problem they once could have solved easily, patients became "dazed, agitated, anxious, started to fumble; a moment before amiable, they became sullen, evasive, and exhibited temper" (Goldstein, 1948). On the other hand, the "therapeutic" effect in frontal lobotomy could be regarded as a manifestation of a deficit in reaction to stress. In such patients, many of whom were psychotic, responsiveness to disturbing thoughts was altered by the operation. The thoughts themselves did not change—delusions and hallucinations continued—but the anxiety and the protective reactions which they had formerly evoked were markedly dampened.

Region of Destruction—Frontal Lobes

Though symptoms of brain dysfunction such as those described above have been seen in patients with brain injury regardless of the site of the lesion, they have often been associated with frontal lobe damage. This has led to the formulation of a "frontal lobe syndrome." The frontal lobes are the largest neocortical region and much of their tissue, particularly anterior to the motor region, can be removed with little or no disturbance of motor and sensory functions. Bilateral frontal lobe damage can cause subtle alterations in the highest integrative functions without causing disorientation or dysmnesia. Lesions of similar extent elsewhere in the neocortex may produce the same symptom complex but, in addition, are necessarily accompanied by disorders of motility, sensory function, speech, and visual motor function; and the subtle manifestations of disordered thought, which stand alone in frontal lobe lesions, may be overshadowed by the presence of the other, more dramatic symptoms.

Although the intellectual changes which are part of the "frontal lobe syndrome" are not specific, it may be worthwhile to list here those additional changes which characteristically occur when the frontal lobes are damaged. There may be a prominent tendency toward inappropriate jocularity (Witzelsucht) as well as inappropriate ill humor. Emotional "incontinence" occurs, i.e., crying and laughing which often alternate rapidly. Such crying and laughing are both provoked by minimal stimuli and often are not related to feelings of sadness or mirth. Indeed, a dampening of subjective emotionality is also characteristic. Dulled responsiveness may lead to poor self-control, inability to understand the consequences of actions, and an inability to orient actions to the social and ethical standards of the community. When lesions are extensive, dulling may give way to torpor and apathy and sometimes to a state of "akinetic mutism" in which the patient will not respond to spoken commands or even to painful stimuli but will lie still, speechless, with open eyes. The patient looks awake and, therefore, is not considered to be in coma yet has little more cognitive function than a comatose person.

Somewhat more specific for frontal lobe disease are motor signs. When the motor portions of the frontal lobe are involved, in particular areas 4 and 6 or their many subcortical connections, motor paralysis may develop. In addition, a form of increased muscle tone known as "gegenhalten" may develop. This is also called "counterpull" and is manifested by semivoluntary resistance which the patient offers increasingly to passive movement of his limbs. When the examiner attempts to extend the patient's elbow, for example, the patient will resist and his resistance will increase as the elbow is extended farther. Forced grasping may be seen in response to tactile stimulation of the patient's palm by the examiner's fingers. When the examiner attempts to extend the patient's fingers while disengaging his own from the patient's grip, he may encounter counterpull.

Various forms of gait disorder may result from frontal lobe damage. One type that is quite similar to cerebellar ataxia may be seen with frontal lobe lesions and presumably reflects the many connections of the frontal lobe with the pons and cerebellum. Apraxia of gait may lead to loss of the ability to stand and walk or even to sit steadily despite well-coordinated movement of the limbs. A form of "marche à petit pas" that resembles the small-stepped gait usually associated with Parkinson's disease may be seen. Increased flexor tone caused by frontal damage ultimately may lead to paraplegia in flexion.

Area 8 of the frontal lobes controls voluntary conjugate eye movements. Stimulation of area 8 causes the eyes to deviate conjugately to the opposite side. Destruction of area 8 leads to deviation of the eyes conjugately to the side of the lesion; however, this is a temporary phenomenon seen mainly in the first days and weeks following acute lesions. During convulsive seizures the head and eyes characteristically turn away from the lesion, and during the postictal phase, they deviate back again toward the lesion.

Parietal Lobe Syndromes and
Language Functions

Like frontal lobe dysfunction, parietal lobe disease gives rise to
rather nonspecific symptoms. Many of the deficits seen with parietal injuries may also result from lesions elsewhere in the brain and
from diseases which involve the brain diffusely. In general, patients
with parietal disease are poor observers, lack an awareness of their

Table 4-1

Some Neurologic Deficits
Seen with Parietal Lobe Damage*

Tactile Dysfunction
"Primary": Hemihypalgesia for touch, pain, heat, and cold
"Cortical": Astereognosis, Agraphesthesia, Extinction on simultaneous bilateral stimulation, Two-point discrimination loss, Position
sense deficit with pseudoathetosis, Sensory ataxia.

Motility Disturbance
Apraxia for learned activities (following commands) or automatic
acts (walking), Gegenhalten, Perseveration, Echopraxia.
Ataxia
Muscular wasting

Constructional Apraxia

Gerstmann Syndrome: Finger Agnosia, Dyscalculia, Right-Left Disorientation, Agraphia

Disordered Body Image
Unilateral neglect
Anosognosia
Denial

Visual Defects
Cortical blindness
Anton's syndrome (blindness with confabulation)
Hemianopia
Distortions: Macropsia, Micropsia, Obliquity, Drifting, Alexia

* Critchley, 1953

deficits and perform variably on psychological tests from day to day. Lesions of the dominant hemisphere usually give rise to disturbances of speech, and lesions of the nondominant hemisphere produce gnostic deficits, faulty corporeal awareness, and defective visual-spatial conceptualization. When such deficits are seen in patients who are not grossly disoriented, or dysmnesic, parietal lobe dysfunction should be suspected. The deficits produced by parietal lobe disease have been considered fully in Critchley's classic mono-

Table 4-2

Origin of Some "Parietal"-Type
Deficits in Single Retrorolandic Lesions*

	Hemisphere	Lobe(s) Mainly Involved
Apraxia		
Constructional	R > L 4:1	Parietal
Dressing	R > L 5:1	Parietal
Agnosia		
Somatognosia		
Denial of half of body opposite lesion	R	Parietal
Finger agnosia (bilat.)	L > R 6:1	Parietal, espec. supramarginal and angular gyri.
Visual Agnosia		
Neglect of space on side opposite lesion	R > L 10:1	Parietal
Nonrecognition of faces	R > L 3:1	Parietal
Nonrecognition of objects, pictures, colors	L	Occipital or post-temporal
Numbers not correctly placed	L > R 3:1	Parietal
Alexia	L	Temporal-Occipital Parietal
Agraphia	L	Temporal-Parietal Occipital
Acalculia	L > R 3:1	Temporal or Parietal

Aphasia

Fluent

Wernicke (poor comprehension, poor repetition)	L	Temporal-Parietal
Conduction (good comprehension, poor repetition)	L	Parietal-Temporal
Anomic-Amnestic (good comprehension, good repetition)		(a) Widespread brain disease
		(b) Recovery from other forms of aphasia
		(c) Also L Parietal (angular gyrus) L Posterior Temporal
Nonfluent (Motor)	L**	Frontal, Temporal, Parietal, Rolandic

* Based on Hécaen (1962) and Geshwind (1971)
** R in a minority of sinistrals

graph (1953). His categorization of abnormality is summarized in Table 4-1. Table 4-2 indicates some of the variability in the location of single retrolandic lesions which may give rise to "parietal" symptoms.

Language

Because language is a cortical function which is unequally represented between and within the hemispheres, its study promises to provide insights into how cortical functions are organized in the central nervous system. Yet the literature on this subject is complex, confusing, and often contradictory. Part of the problem is methodological and part is conceptual; there has not yet been a complete resolution of the opposing views that cortical functions reside in certain anatomical centers and that the cortex is more or less equipotential.

Methodological Problems

Any student of aphasia confronts at least two methodological problems from the start. The first is inaccuracy in defining the anatomical site of the lesion producing aphasia; the second is how to interpret tests for aphasia.

Language is generally considered a uniquely human trait and humans are therefore the only proper subjects for experimentation and research. This means that anatomic correlations with functional deficits must depend in large part upon the study of patients with neurological disease. A variety of lesions can give rise to language deficits in many different ways. Some conditions are progressive and others are not; some tumors produce cerebral edema (causing dysfunction in brain regions far removed from the primary lesion) and others do not. A low-grade glioma and a metastatic lesion may have strikingly different effects even when they share the same anatomical location. Similarly, old scars from trauma or strokes may give rise to seizure activity which can spread to distant brain regions and produce disorders of language which may be incorrectly attributed to the area of the primary lesion. Dominant or left hemispheric strokes sustained in early childhood produce disorders of language quite different from those that follow strokes in adults. Many studies of structure-function correlation in aphasia following traumatic injuries have been based upon a presumed area of brain injury as calculated from a missile trajectory, though distant or contralateral effects of trauma cannot be ruled out before a full pathologic investigation is made (Russell and Espir, 1961). Even when a full pathologic examination has been performed, some investigators have concentrated upon one aspect of a lesion and disregarded others. For example, Broca attributed aphasia to lesions of the frontal operculum and the immediately adjacent cortex. Yet when Marie (1906) restudied Broca's material several years later, he found that the lesions extended into temporal-parietal regions. On other occasions more than one infarct has been found but functional deficits have been attributed to the largest one, and the small lesions in other regions have been regarded as "insignificant" (Nielsen, 1946). The "insignificance" of such small lesions has not been proven.

A rather major difficulty in studying aphasia is the variability of testing methods. The deficits revealed in patients by a specific examination are not necessarily the only deficits they have. In other words, the type and degree of deficit is a function of the type and completeness of testing and in this respect all studies are not comparable. It is not our purpose to discuss aphasia testing in detail. At a minimum, however, clinical evaluation should include tests of the ability to understand spoken and written material, to repeat, to write and to name objects. Notations should be made on the fluency of speech, articulation, and correct use of words in sentences. Nonetheless, even the most thorough testing for aphasia has proven unsatisfactory to some degree in providing a reliable, reproducible method for investigating that complex of factors which determines one's ability to use language. Dissatisfaction with the usefulness of standard testing has provided a stimulus for development of newer psychological and linguistic analyses of language disorders (Jakobson, 1964). No testing system has yet been devised, however, which provides a completely reliable basis for making anatomic-clinical correlations.

Conceptual Barriers

Many of the notions commonly held about the organization of language are inaccurate, though they have been handed down from generation to generation and do bear some relation to the truth. Three such notions are: (a) that the left hemisphere is dominant for language in right-handed persons (dextrals) and the right hemisphere is dominant in left-handed persons (sinistrals); (b) that speech is located in one hemisphere and the organization of language in that hemisphere can be studied by analyzing language deficits in patients who have sustained damage to it; (c) that motor (expressive, nonfluent, or Broca's) aphasia is caused by anterior lesions in the dominant hemisphere while sensory (receptive, fluent, or Wernicke's) aphasia is caused by posterior lesions in the dominant hemisphere and anomic (nominal or amnestic) aphasia may result from temporal lobe lesions in the dominant hemisphere.

ASSUMPTION (a) *There is left speech dominance in dextrals and vice-versa.* There is no question that speech is represented in the left hemisphere in virtually all dextrals. In countless instances, destruction of the left hemisphere in dextrals by tumors, strokes, trauma, or surgery has resulted in aphasia. Destruction of the right hemisphere, on the other hand, virtually never causes serious persistent speech problems in otherwise normal right-handed adults. Still, amytal injections of the right carotid by the Wada technique in epileptic dextrals have been reported to cause speech arrest in 5 of 48 cases (Milner et al., 1964). Thus, right cerebral contributions to speech in some dextrals cannot be entirely discounted, though it is conceivable that in these cases some amytal entered the left circulation.

The situation in sinistrals is more complex. Ettlinger and his associates (1956) found left cerebral speech dominance in 7 of 10 sinistrals. By using intracarotid amytal injections, Milner et al. (1964) found that roughly two-thirds of 44 sinistrals or ambidextrous patients had speech function localized in the left hemisphere. Only in sinistrals with a history of damage to the left hemisphere early in life was speech represented on the right side in the majority of patients (18 of 27). Nonetheless, a minority (20-30 per cent) of normal left-handed individuals are right cerebral dominant for speech and to this degree at least handedness does correlate with hemispheric speech localization. Hécaen and Angelergues (1962) studied 59 sinistrals with unilateral, postrolandic lesions in either the right or the left hemisphere. They also found that left hemispheric lesions more often caused aphasia but noted that language disorders were less serious than in dextrals, had a better prognosis for recovery and, despite their posterior location, tended to be expressive rather than receptive in nature.

ASSUMPTION (b) *Speech is localized in one hemisphere.* There is evidence that the speech function potential of the two hemispheres is equal early in life. It seems that both hemispheres participate as

speech develops in the second and third year of life and that lateralization develops afterward. Thus, destruction of the left or right
hemisphere during the first years of life usually does not prevent
the ultimate development of speech unless there is severe retardation as well; nor does subsequent surgical removal of the damaged
hemisphere cause deterioration of speech (Basser, 1962). Furthermore, damage to either hemisphere in young children who are beginning to speak when brain damage occurs is equally likely to
result in a temporary loss of speech. The bulk of present evidence
indicates that sometime in the middle portion of the first decade
major speech functions become established in the left hemisphere
in most individuals and permanent aphasia is likely to result from
left hemispheric damage thereafter.

The completeness and permanence of the lateralization of
speech in normal adults has long been taken for granted and the
possibility of a contribution to speech by the right hemisphere in
normal dextrals has commonly been overlooked. However, the evidence that the right hemisphere does not participate in speech has
largely rested on an inadequate factual basis, i.e., that destruction
of the right hemisphere does not disturb speech. In fact, stimulation of the right hemisphere may cause vocalization or alter speech
(Penfield and Roberts, 1959), and destruction of the right hemisphere may occasionally result in a certain hesitancy of speech or
other temporary speech deficits.

The contribution of the minor hemisphere to speech has been
investigated by Gazzaniga and Sperry (1967) in patients whose
cerebral hemispheres were functionally separated by commisural
sections. Testing each hemisphere independently, they found that
information perceived by the minor (right) hemisphere could not
be communicated in speech or writing and that complex calculation likewise appeared to be solely a function of the major (left)
hemisphere. Nonetheless, the minor hemisphere showed considerable ability to comprehend written and spoken language, though
less than the major hemisphere. These experiments suggest that in

individuals with intact left hemispheric speech function, the right hemisphere may make some contribution to the understanding of language but is incapable of producing it.

The most impressive evidence of right hemispheric participation in adult language function has recently been presented by Kinsbourne (1971), who studied three right-handed men that suffered left hemispheric strokes which caused aphasia. All were able to speak a little at the time of testing and one had shown considerable improvement, but speech in all three was markedly impaired. Intracarotid injections of amytal caused complete speech arrest when the right carotid was injected but not when the left carotid was injected. It thus appears that whatever speech these patients retained or recovered after they sustained left hemispheric damage originated not in the remaining undamaged portion of the left hemisphere, but rather in the right hemisphere. This is a remarkable demonstration, for it casts great doubt on the validity of some of our most cherished assumptions in the study of language.

It has commonly been implied that dysphasic language in adults with left hemispheric lesions originates in the remaining intact portions of the left hemisphere and that recovery from aphasia is a result of recovered function in partly damaged left hemispheric cells or of recruitment of other previously unused language circuits in the left hemisphere. On the basis of the Kinsbourne study, it appears likely that dysphasic language is largely right hemispheric and that recovery from aphasia depends largely on how completely the right hemisphere can redevelop language skills (i.e., take over the motor language apparatus in the brainstem). The participation of the right hemisphere in dysphasic speech may well be the reason that the various forms of aphasia correlate as incompletely as they do with the anatomic locus of the lesion. Clinical testing of aphasics, in other words, is at least as much a measure of right hemispheric adequacy as it is of left hemispheric damage. The results of Kinsbourne's study provide a good reason for our relative inability to correlate aphasia with anatomical pathology.

Assumption (c) THE QUALITY OF APHASIA HAS LOCALIZING VALUE IN PLACING A CEREBRAL LESION. Neurologists have for a century been intrigued by the possibility of identifying the locus of a cerebral lesion by psychological tests. The goal has been elusive though, and for those who are trying to develop ever more sensitive tests, Monrad-Krohn's caveat still has force: "Nothing can be gained by an untimely anticipation of an anatomical-clinical correspondence, which no doubt exists, but the details of which still for the greater part remain unknown. Until the necessary knowledge has been gathered, all we can do is to avoid muddying the problem in question" (1958).

Most neurologists, nevertheless agree that large anterior lesions are likely to produce disturbances of articulation, hemiparesis, and a form of aphasia in which the patient speaks slowly and with great effort, using single words in a telegraphic style. There is little speech and sentence structure is poor. This form of expressive (motor) aphasia can be seen when the patient's understanding of written and spoken language is largely intact. Even in expressive aphasia, however, there is usually some receptive component to the deficit.

Large posterior lesions are less likely to cause hemiparesis and more likely to cause a disturbance in comprehension. Aphasic speech in such patients may be fairly well articulated but often there is some defect of articulation. Such speech is fluent in the sense that long phrases and sentences with some grammatical structure are used even when words are incorrect and disorganized.

Comprehension and articulation may be normal in amnestic (anomic) aphasia. Patients with amnestic aphasia cannot remember the names of objects. While this may often be seen in patients with temporal lobe damage, it is quite nonspecific and is encountered in patients with dementia, metabolic encephalopathy or lesions elsewhere in the brain.

Though many have tried, it is not clear that much more can be usefully said about anatomic-clinical correlation in aphasia.

Synthesis

Two opposing theories about aphasia had developed by the beginning of the twentieth century and are still maintained. According to one, language is a property of cortical centers which have particular functional significance. Destruction of these centers, of association fibers between them or of projection fibers from them, it is believed, will result in predictable forms of aphasia. According to the other theory, aphasia results from the interruption of widespread circuits within and between the hemispheres. The locus of the lesion is considered less important in determining the speech deficit than the adequacy of the remaining circuits. It seems to us that the latter view is closer to the truth.

The classic work of Penfield and Roberts (1959) provided evidence that supports the second theory. During operations on epileptic patients whose seizures had been impossible to control with medications alone, they stimulated and excised virtually all areas of the cortex which have a role in speech. Stimulation in either hemisphere produced vocalization, arrest of speech, and disordered language. The areas removed in these and other studies that followed have included the parieto-temporal region, the supplementary motor area and Broca's area. Excision of each area has produced only temporary aphasic disturbances as long as the remainder of the brain was intact. These studies indicated that the temporo-parietal region is the most important region for language function, followed by Broca's area. Other regions, such as the supplementary motor area, become indispensable only when the major speech areas are damaged.

Hécaen and Angelergues (1964) performed a systematic language study of 214 right-handed patients with left cerebral lesions in frontal, rolandic, parietal, temporal, and occipital regions. They confirmed the central importance of the posterior temporal region (Wernicke zone) in all language functions, even expressive ones and demonstrated the devastating effects upon language when more than one region was involved.

One is led to the conclusion that language has a supple functional organization within the dominant hemisphere and to a great extent between the hemispheres. What leads to the "dominance" of one hemisphere, how dominance is maintained, and how recovery from aphasia occurs is not known. It is not known whether the change in the language potential of the minor hemisphere which occurs in childhood is the result of inactivity of that hemisphere or whether the dominant zone has some active role in the change. The mechanism of dominance may be analogous to the one demonstrated by Hubel and Wiesel (1965) for the visual cortex. If one eye of an infant kitten is occluded for two to three months the visual cortex becomes permanently unresponsive to impulses from that eye, but is normally responsive to impulses from the unoccluded eye. When both eyes are occluded for two or three months and then tested, the visual cortical cells are still responsive to visual impulses from both eyes. Thus, it appears that the seeing eye of the monocularly occluded cat either preempts all the dendritic connections of the visual cortex or inhibits (suppresses) impulses which come from the eye which had been occluded. This experiment, of course, is analogous to the phenomenon which in humans is known as amblyopia ex anopsia (see Introduction).

In our view, the development of right handedness is part of the process by means of which the left hemisphere becomes dominant for speech and other functions. The fact that major speech functions reside in the left hemisphere of most sinistrals indicates that the two functions—handedness and speech—are independent. Yet the state of left handedness implies that the right hemisphere is not completely subordinate to the left and in such individuals it appears that the speech dominance of the left hemisphere is not as well developed as it is in dextrals. This is manifested by the less serious and less permanent nature of speech deficits which result from left hemispheric lesions in sinistrals. From Kinsbourne's work, we suspect that the speech potential of the right hemisphere of sinistrals has not been permanently rendered ineffective by the dominant left hemisphere. We hypothesize that the right hemisphere of sinistrals is more able to produce speech after damage to the left than that of dextrals.

Like speech, some other cortical functions are unequally represented in various brain regions. Apraxia, agnosia, acalculia, agraphia, and alexia are symptoms which may result from retro-Rolandic lesions. The literature concerning aphasia is much more extensive than that concerning these symptoms but many of the caveats and principles which exist in relation to the study of the organization of speech seem to apply to these other cortical functions too. Lesions in certain portions of the brain are likely to produce these symptoms and yet this does not prove that the lost functions "reside" in specific centers. For lesions in these regions do not always produce the same constellation of symptoms and recovery can occur even after destructive lesions have been sustained. The mechanism of recovery is not clear and it is not yet known if one or both hemispheres participate. Like aphasia, apraxo-agnostic symptoms in sinistrals are generally less severe and less permanent than in dextrals (Hécaen and Angelergues, 1962).

Apraxia can be defined as an inability to carry out a voluntary act, the nature of which the patient understands, in the absence of paralysis, sensory loss, or ataxia. In dextrals, apraxia of both sides of the body is likely to result from lesions in the posterior left hemisphere, especially the supramarginal gyrus of the parietal lobe. Certain forms of apraxia are more likely to result from right parietal lesions; these include dressing apraxia and constructional apraxia (loss of the ability to copy an arrangement of match sticks).

Agnosia is the failure to perceive the nature and meaning of a sensory stimulus when the sensory pathways conveying it are intact. Visual agnosia is present, for example, when a patient is unable to recognize an object he clearly sees. The inability to recognize objects, pictures and colors is virtually always the result of a lesion in the occipital or posterior-temporal regions of the left hemisphere, but lesions in this region do not always give rise to this form of agnosia. The nonrecognition of faces is likely to be associated with a right parietal lesion, though only a minority of patients with right parietal lesions manifest this sign (Hécaen, 1962).

The Gerstmann syndrome: finger agnosia (inability to name the fingers), agraphia, acalculia, and inability to distinguish between right and left, was once thought to be specific for lesions of the angular gyrus of the left parietal lobe (Gerstmann, 1940). Though the observation is correct that lesions in this region can produce this constellation of symptoms, as well as dyslexia, the left angular gyrus is not a "center" for these functions. Agraphia, acalculia, and alexia may result from left temporal lobe lesions, agraphia and alexia from left occipital lobe lesions, and acalculia may be seen in association with right hemispheric lesions (Hécaen, 1962). This information is summarized in Table 4-2.

Temporal Lobes and Memory

When lesions of the temporal lobes produce cognitive deficits, there may be concomitant psychosis, depression, sexual dysfunction and, rarely, episodic violence. These phenomena have been discussed in the chapter on the limbic system and the section on psychomotor epilepsy. The language deficits which may occur in temporal lobe disease have been discussed above. The temporal lobe also plays a role in memory functions, though the mind's ability to record events, to store, and to recall them cannot be regarded as localized in that region. Recent memory loss is the hallmark of all severe organic brain syndromes, whether they are induced by focal or diffuse disease and it is usually associated with extensive cortical dysfunction. There is no doubt, however, that the medial portions of the temporal lobe and the rest of the limbic system play an especially important role in memory function.

In humans limited bilateral lesions in portions of the limbic system are capable of causing a severe, permanent disturbance of recent memory. This has been repeatedly noted after bilateral hippocampal destruction or after unilateral lesions in patients whose other hippocampus was impaired. That both of the hippocampuses are important for recent memory has been further emphasized by the observation that bilateral destruction of the amygdala, another limbic structure, does not cause any memory deficit. The fornix must play some role in memory since bilateral destruction makes the mental recording of ongoing events and their subsequent recall difficult, but the extent of memory deficit after sectioning of the fornices is not as great as that which is caused by hippocampal lesions (Ojemann, 1966).

Lesions in other areas of the brain can also disrupt memory functioning. Destruction of both dorsomedian thalamic (DMT) and medial pulvinar nuclei causes severe recent memory deficits even when the hippocampus is intact. DMT lesions are now thought to be the major anatomical correlate of recent memory loss in Wernicke's encephalopathy. Previously, lesions in the mammillary bodies had been regarded as the locus of dysmnesia in that condition (Victor et al., 1971). Stimulation of the lateral surface of the temporal lobes, especially the superior temporal gyrus, in neurosurgical patients under local anesthesia has evoked remote memories, chiefly auditory and visual, apparently of long forgotten events. Usually these events have been trivial and not of obvious "psychodynamic significance" (Penfield and Perot, 1963). Removal of the stimulated regions has not obliterated such memories, however, so it would be incorrect to conceive of the temporal cortex as a unique memory storage center.

Delirium

In addition to the size and site of a lesion, the nature of the disease process is important in determining the character of an organic brain syndrome. The organic brain syndromes of acute onset, most of which have a toxic or metabolic etiology, are often characterized by delirium. Delirium is not characteristic of chronic brain syndromes. In addition to disorientation and poor memory, delirium has other features. There is fluctuating awareness with occasional lucid periods and somnolence. Often patients are fearful and irritable and suffer from visual hallucinations. Motor signs commonly encountered in delirium include myoclonus, asterixis, and tremulousness.

It must be emphasized that personality changes and thought disorders of a kind usually associated with schizophrenia or depression

Table 4-3

The Differential Diagnosis of Dementia includes:

Degenerative
Alzheimer
Pick
Huntington's Chorea
Senility

Mechanical
Trauma*
Occult hydrocephalus*
Subdurals*

Metabolic
Hypothyroidism*
Hyponatremia*
Hypercalcemia*
Hypoglycemia*
Porphyria*
Hypoxia*
Wilson's*
Uremia*
Hepatic Coma*
CO_2 Narcosis*

Vascular
Arteriosclerosis
Collagen disease*

Neoplastic
Gliomas*
Meningiomas*

Infectious
Lues*
Abscess*
Chronic meningitis*
Subacute sclerosing panencephalitis
Creutzfeldt Jacob

Exogenous Toxin
Metals*
Bromides*
Alcohol*
Barbiturates*
Belladonna alkaloids*
Organic phosphates*
Hallucinogens*

*Vitamin Deficiency**
especially:
Thiamine*
B_{12}*
B_6*
Niacin*
Folate*

* Potentially reversible by medical or surgical means

may be prominent, presenting symptoms of both the chronic and acute forms of an organic brain syndrome. This is frequently a source of diagnostic confusion; patients with structural neurological diseases or toxic and metabolic abnormalities are often misdiagnosed as schizophrenic, depressed, or hysterical on the basis of their most prominent symptoms. Careful attention to the history and physical examination as well as detailed mental status-testing and appropriate laboratory tests, will minimize such errors. The most important point in avoiding a mistaken diagnosis is the awareness that a differential diagnosis exists and must be considered whenever a thought disorder develops (see p. 73).

The prognosis for organic brain syndromes in adults depends upon their etiology. It is quite clear that the chronic, slowly developing syndromes generally have a poorer prognosis than acute cases, but this is not always so. Most of the diseases that cause brain syndromes are potentially reversible, either by medical or surgical means (Table 4-3). Unfortunately, most demented patients suffer from irreversible, progressive disease processes such as arteriosclerosis or senility. Even in these cases, however, the physician can play a positive role by minimizing the discomfort of the patient and his family through wise counsel and judiciously administered medications. For an excellent discussion of the management of the organic brain syndromes, see Detre and Jarecki (1971).

NEUROPSYCHOLOGICAL TESTING

When deficits are moderate or severe, psychological testing usually serves to confirm the physician's clinical impression, but in cases of mild or questionable brain damage psychological tests can provide clinical information that is not readily apparent to a careful interviewer. Many of these tests can give lateralizing information about the site of a lesion and at times provide precise information as to the progression or regression of signs of intellectual dysfunction. Psychological testing is of most use in the diagnosis of questionable cases, in which questions of lateralization are important for both diagnosis and treatment, as well as in longitudinal studies to document the changes in a disease process.

The major tests used to evaluate organic brain damage are performance tests. Projective tests and personality inventories have been of little use in the study of brain damage. The Wechsler Adult Intelligence Scale (WAIS) is divided into a verbal and performance section. Organic deficit usually manifests itself as the disparity between the verbal scales and the performance scales. One would expect patients with left cerebral lesions to do more poorly on the verbal scales than on the performance tasks (spatial and numerical abilities), while the converse would be true of patients with posterior right-hemisphere lesions (Matarazzo, 1972). The performance scales on the WAIS, in terms of block design, picture arrangement, and the assessment of various memory functions, are similar to the more widely used Halstead Battery. In recent years there has been increased interest in the work of Halstead, who developed a reliable battery of tests to assess patients for brain damage. This battery has been modified to a great extent by Reitan and now is usually called the Halstead-Reitan Battery. The modified form consists primarily of the following tasks: (1) The *category test*, a test of concept formation or abstracting ability in which the patient is asked to apply an abstract principle in a series of objects by size, shape, number position, or brightness in color. This may be looked upon as a variation of the many object sorting tasks that were devised by Goldstein and Sheerer and have been referred to on page 77. (2) The *tactile performance test* in which a blindfolded patient is asked to place blocks of varying geometric shapes in the appropriate space on the board by touch alone. He does this with each hand alone and then with both hands. Then he is asked to draw a diagram of the board from memory. The patient is scored for total time to place the blocks with each hand, with both, and finally for his memory of the task.

(3) A *rhythm test* in which the patient is asked to discriminate between rhythmic beats. (4) A *speech sounds perception test* in which the patient has to compare spoken nonsense words with a printed form. (5) A *finger tapping speed* is measured for each hand. (6) A *time sense test* in which the patient is asked to estimate a period of time. (7) A *trail-making test* which demonstrates the patient's ability to follow numbered sequences randomly distributed on paper. (8) A test for *aphasia*. (9) The *WAIS* and, (10) The *Minnesota Multiphasic Personality Inventory* (MMPI). Using this battery of tests, Reitan (1966) succeeded in discriminating brain-damaged from non-brain-damaged patients. Only 4 per cent of the brain-damaged patients and 14 per cent of a control population were misclassified. The test battery is more successful than the WAIS by itself. Its use has suggested that the more posterior the lesion, the greater the intellectual deficit. This is consistent with the observation that many of the tasks measured by these tests (spatial, numerical, and verbal abilities) involve functions whose neurophysiological circuitry is most heavily concentrated in the temporal-parietal regions. By measuring tactile, visual, and auditory perceptual functions, comprehension and abstracting ability, the Halstead-Reitan battery provides an excellent range of tests to evaluate many aspects of psychomotor functioning that are often disturbed in brain-damaged individuals.

Despite their value, psychological test results must be interpreted with caution. There is a tendency to grant these tests the credibility of a laboratory analysis. In fact, all of the confounding variables which must be taken into account in the clinical evaluation of patients accompany the use of these tests, i.e., the age and previous education of the patients, the presence of a static or changing lesion, the acuteness or chronicity of the lesion, the cooperation of the patient, and so forth.

It is also important to note that a battery of tests evaluating numerous functions is more useful than any single test. Most tests that have been devised to evaluate "organicity," such as the Bender

Gestalt, focus on abilities to perform spatial and perceptual motor tasks and therefore provide less data for making a diagnosis of organic brain syndrome than a group of tests would. Differentiating organic brain syndromes from schizophrenia by psychological testing has proved to be quite difficult. The most pervasive disturbance of thinking evident in brain-damaged patients is their concreteness (inability to abstract). As mentioned before (p. 65) the concreteness manifested by organic patients differs somewhat from that of schizophrenic patients. In brain-damaged patients, concreteness is present consistently rather than intermittently. Intermittent concreteness is more characteristic of schizophrenia. The schizophrenic tends to be more bizarre and idiosyncratic, though "organics" can be quite bizarre. One is also more impressed by the "stimulus boundedness" of patients with organic brain syndromes. This psychological term refers to perseveration that is stimulated by and bound to the most recent verbal or visual cues. Schizophrenics tend to go off on wild tangents of loosely connected thoughts when given a particular cue. Often, however, differences between dementia and "dementia praecox" are subtle, and as yet there has not been enough research on the precise differences between the two conditions to be able to reliably distinguish between them on the basis of psychological tests. In fact, there seem to be more similarities than differences.

ORGANIC BRAIN SYNDROMES IN CHILDREN

Especially at an early age, children have a different response to brain damage than adults. Lateralization and dominance with regard to speech, reading, writing, praxis, and so on are not fully established until several years after birth. After early unilateral injury to either hemisphere, most of these functions become established on the healthy side and surgical removal of the damaged tissue produces no further deficit. Thus, unilateral brain damage in children is less likely to cause permanent loss of speech or the other "lateralized" functions. Large unilateral injuries in infants, however, do tend to produce a more widespread deficit in intellectual abilities than similar injuries in adults. It is not clear why this is so. The older a child at the time of injury, the more likely he is to suffer impairment resembling that of an adult with a similar lesion. The classical cortical dysfunctions which may result from single lesions in adults are seen only in young children who have sustained bilateral cortical damage because these functions have not yet become lateralized. These dysfunctions include dyscalculia, right-left confusion, finger agnosia, constructional apraxia (Hansen, 1963) and aphasia (Landau et al., 1960).

EARLY CHILDHOOD AUTISM

Disorders of speech are the hallmark of early childhood autism, a behavioral syndrome first described by Kanner and often mislabeled "childhood schizophrenia." The syndrome includes speechlessness and an inability to make meaningful patterns out of auditory or visual stimuli. It begins in the first few years of life. Characteristically, the first year of life is marked by feeding difficulties and excessive screaming. Motor developmental milestones are usually somewhat delayed but within the normal range. Social withdrawal, odd behavior, and peculiar affect are usually quite noticeable by the second or third year of life. Autistic children have a marked inability to form human relationships and give a sharp impression of extreme solitariness. The severity of these symptoms varies and those children who develop speech by five years of age have a fair chance of achieving independence in later life. Nearly all those who do not speak by this age require permanent care. Autism is often seen in children who also show strong evidence of neurologic abnormality; it may be associated with phenylketonuria, tuberous sclerosis, and infantile spasms during the first year of life. Many autistic children have multiple cognitive deficits and perhaps half have electroencephalographic abnormalities and/or a history of seizures (Kolvin et al., V & VI, 1971; Rutter, 1966; Schain and Yannet, 1960). The symptoms of autism resemble those of congenital aphasia and some neurologists feel it is often nothing more than that.

About the only feature childhood autism shares with schizophrenia is the term "autism," which is one of Bleuler's fundamental symptoms. Otherwise, the two conditions are very different in age of onset, symptomatology, sex distribution (1:1 in schizophrenia; 4 boys to 1 girl in childhood autism), and the social and intellectual status of the patient's family (high in autism and tending toward low in schizophrenia) (Kolvin et al., III, 1971). The most convincing evidence that the two conditions are not identical is genetic. There is no increase in the prevalence of schizophrenia in the parents or siblings of autistic children. Of 521 sibships of autistic children, only 7 contained more than one affected member (Wing, 1966). As mentioned previously, the prevalence of schizophrenia in first degree relatives of schizophrenics is 10 to 15 per cent.

Kanner (1957) and others have noted anecdotally that the mothers of autistic children were emotionally frigid and gave their autistic children only mechanical care. This had been deemed of etiologic significance until a controlled study of the attitudes of mothers toward child rearing failed to confirm the idea. In this study, carefully matched groups of the mothers of autistic, mongoloid, and normal children (100 mothers in each group) were compared. There was very little difference in traits such as overprotection, acceptance, and rejection (Pitfield, and Oppenheim, 1964). Therefore, it seems likely that the cold parental handling of autistic children, when present, is a response to the child's behavior rather than the cause of it (Kolvin et al., IV, 1971).

The bulk of evidence seems to suggest that autism is not a disease entity itself but rather a behavioral syndrome of childhood that can result from many different disorders of the central nervous system, which cause bilateral dysfunction and defective speech. In these terms, it is not difficult to understand why autistic children often have varying deficits in comprehension, symbolic thinking, and the formation of abstract concepts which reflect variations in the degree of CNS dysfunction and the diseases which cause it. This could easily explain why the pattern of cognitive functioning is often uneven with "islets of intelligence."

One strange aspect of autism is the occasional appearance of an isolated, unusual, and highly developed skill in an autistic child. Such is the case of the "idiot savant" who can tell on what day of the week any date will fall, though he is otherwise incapable of doing simple arithmetic and generally functions at a grossly retarded level. Similarly isolated and abnormally developed skills relating to music, memory, or reading have been described in children who appear to be autistic and retarded (Scheerer et al., 1945). The abilities demonstrated by idiot savants are especially striking because they contrast so vividly with the individuals' low intelligence. Such talents, however, are not seen exclusively in idiot savants but may be encountered in persons of average or above average intelligence.

Hardly any information on the neuropathologic correlates of childhood autism has been published. It is a nonprogressive, nonfatal syndrome and brain biopsies cannot usually be justified. Those few cases which have been autopsied and did not reveal some previously unsuspected progressive neurological disease have shown no changes in the brain which could be detected by inspection or by light microscopy with standard staining techniques. While no morphologic correlates of autism and mental retardation have yet been defined, the severity of the functional disruption in these conditions stands in stark contrast to the lack of morphologic findings. This demonstrates the inadequacy of neuropathological techniques, not the "functional" nature of the condition.

MIMINAL BRAIN DAMAGE

The most common symptoms of minimal brain damage may be described as inappropriate, poorly controlled behavior, shortened attention span, and intellectual deficit (Pincus and Glaser, 1966).

Inappropriate activity may take the form of hyperkinesis in which the child, appearing to be driven by some internal force is constantly on the move, touching and handling objects, often briefly and to no discernible purpose. Such behavior is maximal in anxiety-provoking situations and in unfamiliar surroundings. The term hyperkinesis may often be a misnomer for quantitative analysis of movement is usually lacking. The distinction between a normally "active" child and a "hyperactive" one is largely a matter of clinical impression. Inappropriate activity may also take the form of listlessness, withdrawal, and negativism.

Attention span is often altered, and affected children are unable to focus upon anything for a sustained period. In severe cases the child will respond in rapid succession to any stimulus in his environment with equal intensity. This may be the basis for the frenetic activity so characteristic of the syndrome. Attention span is not merely shortened but inappropriate and unpredictable; attention sometimes becomes riveted upon trivia and at other times seems to be totally absent.

Impulsive, poorly controlled behavior may be destructive when the child rapidly touches and moves objects. It may also involve aggressive acts, tantrums, sexual displays, and verbal outbursts directed at others. Changes in accustomed routine or unfamiliar demands can provoke such outbursts. Some clinicians have observed decreased capacity for spontaneous affectionate behavior and a failure to respond to reprimand or punishment.

The procedures which are most often used to assess the possibility of organic brain damage are a carefully taken medical history, complete physical and neurological examinations, and psychological tests.

School failure caused by intellectual deficits of many varieties is a regular occurrence among children with mild brain damage. These deficits may be generalized or patchy. There is often a history of delayed developmental milestones. Specific difficulty with arithmetic and delayed acquisition of reading and writing skills are common. Learning disabilities may also reflect difficulties in hearing, language comprehension, memory and speech, and in the ability to generalize and classify. Such perceptual limitations may contribute to the difficulties that these children have in controlling their activity. Intelligence quotients may be normal, and sophisticated psychological testing may be necessary to reveal areas of dysfunction and define them. Intelligence, however, is low in general, being in the boderline or defective range in about half of the cases.

The behavioral manifestations of mild brain damage in childhood differ from those of adults and have been carefully studied only in the past 10 to 15 years. The incidence of "minimal brain damage" in children is high; children with this "syndrome" form a large part of the patient population seen in general pediatric clinics as well as by neurologists, child psychiatrists, and psychologists and all other clinicians who deal with learning problems in childhood. There has been increasing awareness among educators of the possibility of organic brain damage in school children and increasing and perhaps inappropriate use of this diagnostic terminology by many who apply it to virtually any kind of behavioral aberration or deviation from norms of academic performance. Many states are organizing programs to assist those children who are designated as having a "neurologic impairment to learning." The use of special educational techniques in such cases has been shown in controlled studies to be helpful (Cruickshank et al., 1961); and these factors call for clarity in diagnosis. Most children with this syndrome have no major sign of neurologic deficit, such as hemiplegia, but many do have minor signs. These include clumsiness, impaired succession movements, excessive synkinesis, motor impersistence, mild involuntary movements of a choreiform nature, inability to perform tandem gait, to stand on either foot, to hop, or, in children of more than seven years of age, to skip. Impairment of stereognosis and graphesthesia and two point discrimination are other common findings.

As virtually all of these physical signs can be seen in younger normal children (less than five years old) many have questioned their significance when found in older children and have viewed the entire syndrome, including minor neurological abnormalities, learning problems, and abnormal behavior as the result of delayed maturation of the nervous system or psychological immaturity. It is true that one cannot predict on the basis of behavior, which children will have minor neurologic signs and vice versa. In addition, no neuropathological basis for the minor neurological signs has been established. The question whether these signs represent organic disease or delayed maturation cannot be resolved without follow-up studies to indicate whether or not the signs disappear as children grow older. The prognosis for minimal brain damage in children depends largely on etiology, but since the etiology is so often in doubt (no completely convincing longitudinal studies have been done), prediction is difficult. In general, the hyperkinetic behavior tends to disappear by adulthood but associated intellectual deficits remain.

O'Neal and Robins (1958) have related childhood problems to adult psychiatric status in a 30-year retrospective study of 150 subjects who had been evaluated in childhood but not treated at the St. Louis Municipal Psychiatric Clinic. This group was compared to a control group of 150 individuals of similar age and background who had been seen in nonpsychiatric clinics. A very high rate of sociopathy and psychosis was found in the study group. How many of the disturbed children might have had minimal brain damage was not indicated; however, since a very high proportion (perhaps 40 to 50 per cent) of children referred to psychiatric clinics and child-guidance clinics do have academic problems and behavior disorders, it might be reasonable to assume that many of the individuals in O'Neals and Robins's study did have the syndrome as children. From this, it might further be assumed that minimal brain damage in childhood increases the risk of developing a psychosis and sociopathic personality later in life.

It has not been clearly demonstrated that drug treatment of hyperkinetic behavior is effective. Anticonvulsants are, of course, used for seizures, but their effects on the behavioral disturbance may vary. Sedating drugs and one excellent anticonvulsant, phenobarbital, often seem to exacerbate hyperkinetic behavior. Anticonvulsants usually do not alleviate behavioral disorders in children with abnormal electroencephalograms but without clinical seizures. Alerting drugs such as the amphetamines and methylphenidate seem to calm children and help them organize their behavior apparently by reducing fluctuations in vigilance and alertness and by increasing attention span. Chlorpromazine may have a tranquilizing effect and is also known to reduce the severity of choreiform movement disturbances. Chlordiazepoxide and its analogs, such as diazepam, have been used with similarly inconsistent results.

REFERENCES

Basser, L. S.   Hemiplegia of early onset and the faculty of speech with special reference to the effects of hemispherectomy. Brain 85: 427, 1962.

Chapman, L. F. and H. G. Wolff.   The cerebral hemispheres and the highest integrative functions of man. Arch. Neurol. 1: 357, 1959.

Columbia-Greystone Associates. In F. A. Mettler, ed., Selective Partial Ablation of the Frontal Cortex. Paul B. Hoeber. Harper and Brothers, New York, 1949.

Critchley, M.   The Parietal Lobes. Edward Arnold, London, 1953.

Cruickshank, W. M., F. A. Bentzen, F. H. Ratzeburg, and M. T. Tannhauser.   A Teaching Method for Brain-Injured & Hyperactive Children: A demonstration-pilot study. Syracuse University Press, Syracuse, 1961 (Series 6 Syracuse University Special Education & Rehabilitation Monograph).

Detre, T. P. and H. G. Jarecki.   Modern Psychiatric Treatment. J. B. Lippincott Co., Philadelphia, 1971.

Ettlinger, G., C. V. Jackson, and O. L. Zangwill.   Cerebral dominance in sinistrals. Brain 79: 569, 1956.

Gazzaniga, M. S. and R. W. Sperry.   Language after section of the cerebral commissures. Brain 90: 131, 1967.

Gerstmann, J. Syndrome of finger agnosia, disorientation for right and left, agraphia, and acalculia. Arch. Neurol. Psychiat. 44: 398, 1940.

Geshwind, N. Aphasia. New Eng. J. Med. 284: 654, 1971.

Goldstein, K. After-Effects of Brain Injuries in War: Their Evaluation and Treatment. Grune and Stratton, New York, 1948.

Hansen, E. Reading and writing difficulties in children with cerebral palsy. In: R. C. MacKeith and M. Bax, eds., Minimal Cerebral Dysfunction. 1963 (No. 10 Little Club Clinics in Developmental Medicine), p. 58.

Hécaen, H. Clinical symptomatology in right and left hemisphere lesions. In: V. B. Mountcastle, ed., Interhemispheric Relations and Cerebral Dominance. Johns Hopkins University Press, Baltimore, 1962, p. 215.

――― and P. Angelergues. Localization of symptoms in aphasia. In: Disorders of Language. Little, Brown and Co., Boston, 1964 (Ciba Foundation Symposium), p. 223.

――― and ―――. L'aphasie, l'agnosie chez les gauchers: modalités et fréquence des trouble selon l'hémisphère atteint. Rev. Neurol. 106: 510, 1962.

Jakobson, R. Towards a linguistic typology of aphasic impairments. In: Hécaen and Angelerques, Disorders of Language, p. 21.

Kanner, L. Child Psychiatry. 3rd ed. C. C. Thomas, Springfield, Ill., 1957.

Kinsbourne, M. The minor cerebral hemisphere as a source of aphasic speech. Arch. Neurol. 25: 302, 1971.

Kolvin, I, C. Ounsted, L. M. Richardson, and R. F. Garside. III The family and social background in childhood psychoses. Brit. J. Psychiat. 118: 396, 1971.

―――, R. F. Garside, and J. S. H. Kidd. IV Parental personality and attitude and childhood psychoses. Brit. J. Psychiat. 118: 403, 1971.

―――, C. Ounsted, and M. Roth. V Cerebral dysfunction and childhood psychoses. Brit. J. Psychiat. 118: 407, 1971.

―――, M. Humphrey, and A. McNay. VI Cognitive factors in childhood psychoses. Brit. J. Psychiat. 118: 415, 1971.

Landau, W. M., R. Goldstein, and F. R. Kleffner. Congenital aphasia: a clinico-pathologic study. Neurology 10: 915, 1960.

Lashley, K. S. Brain mechanisms and intelligence. University of Chicago Press, Chicago, 1929.

Levenson, F. and V. Meyer. Personality changes in relation to psychiatric status following orbital cortex undercutting. Brit. J. Psychiat. 3: 207, 1965.

Marie, P. Revision de la question de l'aphasie: la troisième circon-
volution frontale gauche ne joue aucun rôle spécial dans la fonction du
language. Sem. Med. 26: 241, 1906.

Matarazzo, J. D.   In Wechsler's Measurement and Appraisal of Adult
Intelligence. 5th ed. Williams and Wilkins Co., Baltimore. 1972.

Milner, B., C. Branch, and T. Rasmussen. Observations on cerebral
dominance. In: Hécaen and Angelergues, Disorders of Language, p. 200.

Moniz, E.   Les premières tentatives opératoires dans le traitement de
certaines psychoses. Encéphale 31: 1, 1936.

Monrad-Krohn, G. H.   The Clinical Examination of the Nervous System. Lewis, London, 1958.

Nielsen, J. M.   Agnosia, Apraxia, Aphasia: Their Value in Cerebral
Localization. 2nd ed. P. B. Hoeber, New York, 1946.

Ojemann, R. G.   Correlations between specific human brain lesions
and memory changes: A critical survey of the literature. Neurosci. Res.
Prog. Bull. 4: 1, 1966.

O'Neal, P. and L. N. Robins.   The relationship of childhood behavior
problems to adult psychiatric status: A 30 year followup study of 150
subjects. Am. J. Psychiat. 114: 961, 1958.

Penfield, W. and P. Perot. The brain's record of auditory and visual
experience. Brain 86: 595, 1963.

——— and L. Roberts. Speech and Brain Mechanisms. Princeton
University Press, Princeton, 1959.

Pincus, J. H. and G. H. Glaser.   The syndrome of "minimal brain
damage" in childhood. New Eng. J. Med. 275: 27, 1966.

Pitfield, M. and A. N. Oppenheim.   Child rearing attitudes of mothers of psychotic children. J. Child Psychol. Psychiat. 5: 51, 1964.

Reitan, R. M.   Research program on psychological effects of brain
lesions in human beings. In: N. R. Ellis, ed. International Review of
Research in Mental Retardation. Vol. 1 p. 153, Academic Press, New
York, 1966.

Russell, W. and M. L. E. Espir. Traumatic Aphasia. Oxford University Press, London, 1961.

Rutter, M.   In: J. K. Wing, ed., Early Childhood Autism: Clinical,
Educational and Social Aspects. Pergamon Press, London, 1966, p. 51.

Schain, R. J. and H. Yannet. Infantile autism: an analysis of 50 cases
and a consideration of revelant neurophysiologic concepts. J. Pediat.
57: 560, 1960.

Scheerer, M., E. Rothmann, and K. Goldstein.   A case of "idiot savant": An experimental study of personality organization. Psych. Monographs 58, no. 4, 1945.

Victor, M., R. D. Adams, and G. H. Collins. The Wernicke-Korsakoff Syndrome: A Clinical and Pathological Study of 245 Patients, 82 with Post Mortem Examination. Contemporary Neurology Series #7. F. A. Davis Co., Philadelphia, 1971.

Wiesel, T. N. and D. H. Hubel. Comparison of the effects of unilateral and bilateral eye closure on cortical unit responses in kittens. J. Neurophysiol. 28: 1029, 1965.

Wing, J. K. In: J. K. Wing, ed. Early Childhood Autism, p. 3.

Chapter 5

BIOGENIC AMINES IN MOVEMENT DISORDERS, DEPRESSION, PSYCHOSIS, AND SLEEP

Recent advances in the study of the catecholamines have led to a greater understanding of Parkinson's disease and the biochemical mechanisms of action of drugs which modify its symptoms. Many of the drugs used for Parkinsonism are known to be effective in treating other neurologic and psychiatric conditions, especially chorea, depression, and thought disorders. Combined with clinical experience in using these drugs, the insight into their mechanisms of action provided by basic research has made it possible to construct at least a tentative hypothesis concerning the biochemical abnormalities which may underlie depression, some movement disorders, and some psychoses.

PARKINSON'S SYNDROME

Clinical Features

There are three major clinical features of the Parkinsonian syndrome: tremor, rigidity, and bradykinesia. The *tremor* of Parkinsonism is apparent mainly when the patient is resting or holding sustained postures and is diminished during voluntary movements. For this reason, of the three cardinal symptoms, tremor interferes least with willed body movements. *Rigidity* is a manifestation of increased muscle tone and it is maximal in flexor muscles. This results in the stooped posture with slight flexion of the knees, hips, neck, and elbows so characteristic of Parkinsonism. In practical terms, rigidity means that patients with Parkinsonism must overcome increased tone in antagonistic muscles in order to move, and extensor functions are especially limited. The extra effort needed to move is often interpreted by the patient as weakness but individual muscle testing frequently provides little evidence of loss of strength. The *bradykinesia* of Parkinsonism is best defined as a disability in initiating and sometimes arresting movement. Patients with Parkinson's disease may have great difficulty carrying out associated or spontaneous movements such as swinging the arms while walking, and often it takes them a few seconds to begin walking. Not infrequently they will run into a wall or a door in order to stop.

Other clinical features of Parkinsonism which relate to the three cardinal symptoms are: expressionless features, a feeling of weakness and of being slowed down, flattening and weakness of the voice, micrographia, marche à petit pas, cogwheel rigidity, and festinating gait. Oily seborrheic skin, excessive salivation, constipation, difficulty focusing the eyes, and sleep disturbances suggested autonomic dysfunction, namely parasympathetic overactivity, in Parkinsonism many years before much was known about the pathogenesis of the condition.

Parkinson's syndrome has many causes. The most common one today is probably the use of tranquilizing medications such as the phenothiazines, other major tranquilizers, or rauwolfia alkaloids. The idiopathic, postencephalitic and arteriosclerotic causes of Parkinson's syndrome are also fairly common. In these forms, the disease affects people over fifty years of age and is seldom familial. The etiology of idiopathic Parkinsonism is in doubt but the idea that a slow virus could be responsible has gained wide currency. Other rare causes of Parkinson's syndrome are carbon monoxide poisoning, manganese intoxication, hypocalcemia, and degenerative diseases of the nervous system in which Parkinsonian features are seen. In this discussion, we will be concerned mostly with drug-induced and idiopathic syndromes.

It is not usually difficult to distinguish Parkinsonism from other neurological disorders. The condition most easily confused with Parkinsonism is depression. In depression, generalized weakness, slowing down of movement, expressionless features, weakened voice, small steps, diminution of spontaneous movements, constipation, and sleep disturbances are seen. All these symptoms are similar to features of Parkinsonism. Many clinicians have claimed that depression to some degree is virtually always seen in patients with Parkinson's disease. This has been disputed, but it is true that most patients with Parkinson's disease do look depressed, especially at rest.

The histopathology of idiopathic and postencephalitic Parkinson's disease appears minor, giving one little indication of the clinical severity of the disorder. Even though a person may be virtually imprisoned in his body, almost unable to move, the neuropathology of Parkinsonism may not be very dramatic. The substantia nigra is the primary site of lesions. While other regions may be affected too, this is the only part of the nervous system where lesions always occur. The changes seen in the substantia nigra are a disappearance of neurons and a displacement into extracellular space of the pigment ordinarily present in the neurons of this region. In addition, some reactive gliosis is seen. Peculiar cytoplasmic inclusion bodies, called Lewy bodies, occasionally appear in the neurons of the substantia nigra.

Physiology

The neurophysiological defects in Parkinson's disease have been difficult to define exactly but a sensible theory has been put forward by Carmen (1966). Lesions of the substantia nigra, according to this theory, produce movement problems because of a loss of nigro-striatal influence. The substantia nigra is conceived as having an inhibitory effect on the globus pallidus which, when unopposed, has an excitatory effect upon motor movements that results in tremor. This excitation is mediated mainly by pathways which travel from the globus pallidus to the ventral anterior and ventral lateral nuclei of the thalamus. These nuclei in turn project to the motor cortex and influence movement. In other words, Carmen has suggested an ascending pathway: the substantia nigra inhibits the globus pallidus, the globus pallidus sends messages to the thalamus, the thalamus transmits these messages to the motor cortex. In Parkinson's disease the messages are incorrect because of the tissue change in the substantia nigra. Destruction of the globus pallidus was long ago shown by Cooper (1968) to relieve the tremor of Parkinsonism. A modification of the operation which has been more effective involves destruction of portions of the thalamus, the way station in the transmission of incorrect afferent information to the motor cortex. Many movement disorders that may result from dysfunction of the basal ganglia can be relieved by placing lesions in this region of the thalamus. Intention tremor which presumably arises from a disorder of the dentate nucleus of the cerebellum, hemiballismus which is caused by lesions in the subthalamic nucleus, and dystonia which sometimes results from abnormalities of the putamen, may be abolished by thalamic lesions. The advantage of thalamotomy over previous operations which destroyed the cortico-spinal pathways is that while both procedures abolish excessive abnormal movement, the former does not produce paralysis but the latter always does.

This operation is not the ultimate answer to Parkinson's disease because beyond the obvious risks of operating on elderly people, and the fact that unilateral lesions are not sufficient to treat an essentially bilateral disease, thalamotomy does not abolish bradykinesia and has a disappointingly mild effect upon rigidity. It has been very effective in abolishing tremor, but tremor is the least disabling of the three major symptoms of Parkinson's disease. The failure of thalamic lesions to ameliorate all the symptoms of Parkinson's disease suggests that Carmen's theoretical model of the pathophysiology underlying the condition is oversimplified and possibly incorrect.

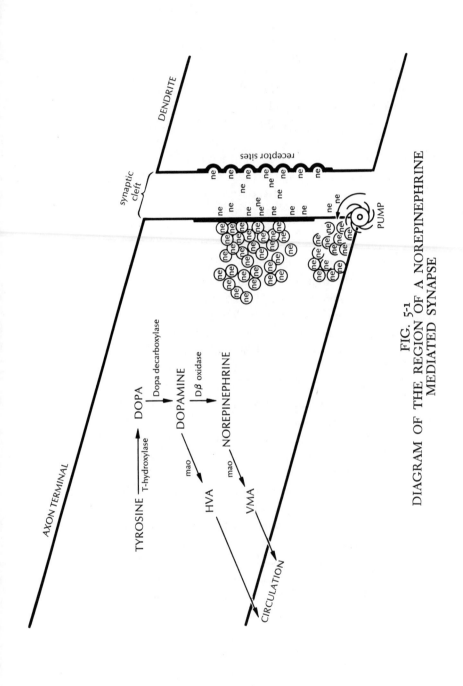

FIG. 5-1
DIAGRAM OF THE REGION OF A NOREPINEPHRINE
MEDIATED SYNAPSE

Biochemistry

Biochemical studies in the last decade have offered a promising approach to full understanding of Parkinson's disease and other related conditions. One of the initial breakthroughs was the demonstration that certain neurons in the central nervous system contain catecholamines (dopamine, norepinephrine) and serotonin. It was further demonstrated that these amine-containing neurons are not uniformly distributed. Serotonin is found primarily in the cells of the median raphé and hippocampus; norepinephrine reaches its highest concentrations in the hypothalamus and the highest concentrations of dopamine are found in the caudate nucleus and putamen, then the globus pallidus and substantia nigra (Cooper, Bloom and Roth, 1970). In postmortem studies of the brains of patients with Parkinson's disease, dopamine and its principal metabolite, homovanillic acid, were found to be reduced to one-tenth of their normal concentration in the basal ganglia (Hornykiewicz, 1966). These findings have led to the development of a rational and highly effective drug treatment for this condition.

Catecholamine Metabolism

The catecholamines, dopamine and norepinephrine, are synthesized from the amino acid, tyrosine, by a series of enzymatic steps (see Fig 5-1). Tyrosine is taken into neurons and hydroxylated through the action of the enzyme tyrosine hydroxylase to DOPA. DOPA, by means of the enzyme dopa-decarboxylase, is converted to dopamine. Dopamine is stored in some neurons (called "dopaminergic") in which it is thought to be a neurotransmitter. Dopaminergic neurons are concentrated in the basal ganglia. In those neurons which store norepinephrine ("noradrenergic") the presumed transmitter substance is norepinephrine. In noradrenergic neurons, dopamine acts as a precursor of norepinephrine. By the action of dopamine beta oxidase, norepinephrine is synthesized from dopamine. Though widely distributed, noradrenergic neurons are highly concentrated in the hypothalamus.

In the conversion of tyrosine to dopamine or norepinephrine, it has been established that the action of tyrosine hydroxylase is the rate-limiting step. This means that reduction in the activity of this enzyme reduces proportionally the production of both dopamine and norepinephrine. Inactivation of other enzymes in this pathway does not lead to proportional decreases in the production of the catecholamines. That tyrosine hydroxylase activity is inhibited by the catecholamines, suggests a negative feedback mechanism whereby the production of norepinephrine and dopamine provokes a decline in their production. Direct nerve stimulation has been shown to accelerate norepinephrine biosynthesis, presumably by eliciting release of the transmitter, and thus depleting the pool of norepinephrine within the neuron which inhibits the enzyme activity.

An analogous set of reactions occurs in the formation of the indoleamines. By similar steps, tryptophane is taken up by "serotonergic" neurons and is converted to 5-hydroxytryptophane and then to 5-hydroxytryptamine (5HT or serotonin). The rate-limiting step in this series is the one catalyzed by tryptophane hydroxylase. In all tissues where catecholamines and indoleamines are found, they are located within highly specialized subcellular particles. In the central nervous system, these particles are called synaptic vesicles and they are concentrated at axon terminals (see Fig. 5-1). Stimulation of the axon causes release of the contents of these vesicles into the synaptic cleft, where they then activate receptor sites on the dendritic membrane and thus accomplish impulse transmission from cell to cell.

Catecholamines undergo a rather complex fate. One portion is metabolized by catechol-O-methyl transferase (COMT) and another by monamine oxidase (MAO). MAO also degrades serotonin. Enzymatic degradation, however, plays a relatively minor role in the inactivation of these transmitter amines. The major portion of released neurotransmitter is taken up again by the neuron. This process, called reuptake, depends upon an active pumping mechanism which rapidly and economically terminates the action of the released transmitter. Reuptake is the major mechanism by which indoleamines, as well as catecholamines are removed from the receptor sites. At cholinergic sites, on the other hand, the major mechanism for the inactivation of acetylcholine is enzymatic rather than a reuptake process.

Once the released amine is taken up by the axon, it is stored again in vesicles. Few amine-containing vesicles release their contents during nerve stimulation; thus, most of the amine within the axon terminals is essentially in an inactive form. This allows us to roughly equate "reuptake" with "inactivation" when speaking of transmitter amines.

Monamine oxidase, which is present within the amine containing axons, serves to inactivate any excess catecholamines that may leak out of the storage vesicles. As a result of MAO action, by-products of the amines are formed and then excreted via blood and spinal fluid and finally the kidneys. These by-products include vanillymandelic acid (VMA), a breakdown product of norepinephrine, and homovanillic acid (HVA), a breakdown product of dopamine. Five-hydroxyindoleacetic acid (5HIAA) is the major breakdown product of serotonin. These by-products have been measured in spinal fluid and urine and have provided information concerning the role of catecholamines in neurological and psychiatric diseases.

Several groups of drugs are effective in treating Parkinson's disease. The most effective, in order of their chronological introduction into the pharmacopoeia for treatment of Parkinson's disease, are: (1) belladonna alkaloids (anticholinergics), (2) levo dihydroxyphenylalanine (L-dopa), and (3) amantadine. Other drugs that have some beneficial effect in patients with Parkinsonism are the amphetamines, the monamine oxidase inhibitors (MAOI), and the tricyclic mood elevators. Other medications induce or exacerbate Parkinson's syndrome. The rauwolfia alkaloids (reserpine), the phenothiazines and the other major tranquilizers (butyphenones, etc.), administered in high doses to neurologically normal individuals can produce all the symptoms of Parkinsonism.

Treatment of Parkinson's Syndrome and the Biochemical Basis of Drug-Action: Anticholinergics

Because of the apparent parasympathetic overactivity in patients with Parkinson's disease, they used to be given anticholinergic drugs such as scopolamine (Hyoscine) and stramonium. These have been supplanted by synthetic compounds such as trihexyphenidyl (Artane) and benztropine (Cogentin), which are effective in reducing salivation and rigidity. Bradykinesia is occasionally alleviated by these agents, but tremor is largely unaffected. In idiopathic Parkinson's disease the best result one can expect from these agents is a 20 to 30 per cent improvement in 60 to 70 per cent of patients (Goodman and Gilman, 1970). The phenothiazine-induced Parkinsonism responds very differently, however. Immediate remission of symptoms occurs after intravenous injection of an anticholinergic drug or even after injection of certain antihistamines with anticholinergic properties such as diphenhydramine (Benadryl). Total remission of Parkinsonian symptoms is the rule when anticholinergics are administered orally to psychiatric patients who are receiving high doses of phenothiazines or related major tranquilizers.

The demonstration of low dopamine levels in postmortem studies of the brains of Parkinsonian patients has led to the "balance" theory of Parkinsonism and its treatment (Van Woert et al., 1972; Weintraub and Van Woert, 1971). According to this theory, cholinergic and adrenergic brain mechanisms must be in balance. In Parkinsonism the adrenergic mechanisms are weakened by loss of dopamine. The anticholinergic drugs reduce cholinergic activity and thus restore a balance that leads to clinical improvement. Evidence supporting this theory has been adduced from experiments that demonstrated a worsening of Parkinsonism when the centrally acting antiacetylcholinesterase medication, physostigmine (Eserine), is injected. This deterioration is conceived as resulting from the increased cholinergic activity induced by physostigmine. Although attractive, the balance theory does not offer a ready explanation for the difference in the effectiveness of anticholinergic drugs with idiopathic and phenothiazine-induced Parkinsonism. Recently, it was found that the anticholinergic drugs are potent inhibitors of dopamine reuptake into synaptosomes isolated from rat corpus striatum (Coyle and Snyder, 1969). This may well be the major site of action of the anticholinergic drugs used to treat Parkinsonism. By reducing reuptake, these drugs may lead to an accumulation of dopamine in the extracellular region, thus prolonging its opportunity to act at receptor sites on the dendritic membrane. In idiopathic Parkinson's disease, however, since there is little dopamine in the brain and therefore little is released into the synaptic cleft, the anticholinergic drugs would be expected to have little effect.

The phenothiazines are thought to act primarily by competitively blocking the postsynaptic receptor sites of the transmitter amines. In animals that have been treated with large doses of phenothiazines, total brain dopamine levels are not reduced and in fact may be elevated. Thus, the amount of dopamine that is released from the axon by nerve stimulation is much greater in phenothiazine-induced Parkinsonism than it is in idiopathic Parkinson's disease. Inactivation of the reuptake mechanism in phenothiazine-induced Parkinsonism would lead to a marked elevation in the concentration of dopamine in the synaptic cleft and would be expected to overcome the competitive block formed by phenothiazines. Thus, it seems likely that the anticholinergics may modify Parkinsonism primarily through their effect on the catecholamine inactivation system; this theory offers the best available explanation of the differential efficacy of anticholinergics in the treatment of idiopathic and phenothiazine-induced Parkinsonism.

Although anticholinergic drugs are of little use in neurology and psychiatry beyond the treatment of Parkinsonism, some of their other effects should be noted. In toxic doses they may produce nightmares, agitation, and delirium. The mental state that can be produced by the anticholinergic compounds may strikingly resemble that which is seen in schizophrenia. The drugs may give rise to loose associations, auditory hallucinations and inappropriate affect in people who have normal orientation and memory. The dose of an anticholinergic drug does not have to be unusually high to induce psychosis as there seems to be a large element of individual sensitivity to these drugs. For this reason, it is wise to start anticholinergic medication with very small doses to be sure that patient can tolerate them. The delirium caused by these drugs is usually associated with tachycardia, fever, dilated pupils, flushing of the skin, visual hallucinations, and disorientation, but these signs may not be prominent. When high doses of anticholinergic compounds are used in combination with phenothiazines for the treatment of schizophrenia, they may occasionally make the schizophrenic symptoms worse.

Theoretically, the belladonna compounds might have some antipressant action (cf. p. 149) as they reduce reuptake of dopamine. They are not known, however, to have any antidepressant effect. Yet, their effect upon depression is apparently not different from that of an effective antidepressant, imipramine. In a study of the treatment of depression performed in 1965, comparing imipramine with an active placebo (atropine), no difference between imipramine and the placebo was found (Tucker, unpublished). Atropine was chosen for this study because the cholinergic side effects such as dry mouth, constipation and visual blurring are the same as those produced by imipramine. In the light of many subsequent studies indicating the great usefulness of imipramine in the treatment of depression the question can be raised whether belladonna compounds might in fact have an antidepressant effect. There are some shreds of evidence that this is so. Scopolamine has long been known to have a "tranquilizing" effect when used preoperatively and often relieves a patient's agitation. In therapeutic doses it normally causes drowsiness and euphoria. Its major drawback is that it may occasionally produce excitement and delirium in doses in the normal therapeutic range (Goodman and Gilman, 1970).

L-Dopa

The suspicion and final demonstration that dopamine deficiency in the basal ganglia is the basic chemical defect in Parkinson's disease led to clinical trials with agents likely to replenish the deficient amine. Because dopamine itself does not cross the blood/brain barrier, the precursor, dopa, first in the racemic form and now in the levo form, has been used. This compound is unquestionably the most effective therapy that has yet been devised for Parkinson's disease. The drug primarily reduces rigidity and bradykinesia and though less effective for treating tremor, it basically helps this symptom also. Roughly 80 per cent of all patients on L-dopa experience 60 to 70 per cent improvement. In order to be effective in Parkinson's disease, large doses of L-dopa must be used; most patients do not experience a significant beneficial effect unless they are taking between 3 and 8 grams per day by mouth. As a result, side effects are extremely common. Of these, the most relevant to our discussion are movement disorders and emotional changes.

In about half the patients treated with L-dopa involuntary movements, ranging from mild and fleeting to severe and prolonged, develop. Choreiform movements of the legs, arms, and face are often seen and these involuntary movements can become so severe that they may resemble hemiballismus. The development of such movements is definitely linked to improved control of Parkinsonism. In some cases it is impossible to relieve the major symptoms of Parkinson's disease without inducing choreiform movements (Cotzias et al., 1969).

About 10 per cent of all patients being treated for Parkinson's disease with L-dopa experience changes in their mental state which are occasionally severe enough to warrant discontinuation of the medication. These changes include confusion with paranoid features, frank psychotic breaks, hypomania, agitation, and aggressive-impulsive behavior. L-dopa aggravates psychosis when given to schizophrenics (Yaryura-Tobias et al., 1970). The mechanism by which L-dopa induces such mental aberrations is not at all clear. Hornykiewicz (1970) has studied the brains of L-dopa-treated Parkinsonian patients at autopsy. He found that dopa therapy only slightly increases concentrations of dopamine in the brain tissues. Though elevated in comparison with levels found in the brains of untreated patients, dopamine in the brains of treated Parkinsonian patients is still below normal. Brain HVA levels are very high, suggesting a rapid turnover and a high rate of activity in the conversion of dopa to dopamine and then to the breakdown product, HVA. The HVA/DOPA ratio is higher in the basal ganglia than in the temporal cortex and this indicates a higher dopamine turnover rate in the basal ganglia than in the cerebral cortex. The fact that there is no large dopamine accumulation in dopa-treated Parkinsonian patients may indicate either that dopamine is not being stored properly or that it is being too rapidly utilized and metabolized to HVA. Some confirmation for this view was obtained by Barbeau (1970) in studies of the platelets of patients with Parkinson's disease. Finding that platelets took up dopamine normally but released it too quickly, he suggested there might be a generalized tissue defect in Parkinson's disease, i.e., that tissues utilizing dopamine are unable to store it properly.

This relatively simple schema may not explain all the clinical effects of L-dopa, for use of this compound has effects on the other brain amines. L-dopa is known to augment the release of serotonin, and dopamine is taken up into serotonergic neurons during L-dopa therapy. Thus, dopa may to some degree act as a false transmitter at serotonin receptor sites and some of its clinical effects may relate to a relative serotonin deficiency. Exogenously administered L-dopa does not very much increase the amount of norepinephrine in the brain. L-dopa treatment in cats has actually been noted to decrease norepinephrine levels in the hypothalamus. This may be the result of an increase in norepinephrine release induced by dopamine. Thus, the interaction between the indoleamines and catecholamines is highly complex. An excess of one is likely to lead to increased release and possibly to depletion of the others. This complexity renders tentative any simple theory of the mechanism by which L-dopa and other drugs used to treat Parkinsonism produce behavioral and neurological changes.

Amantadine

Amantadine, first introduced as an antiviral agent, was accidently found to have activity against Parkinsonism. Until recently, its mechanism of action was unknown. Many of its side effects are similar to those of the anticholinergic drugs. These include dryness of the mouth, difficulty in focusing vision, insomnia, and psychosis. Nonetheless, the drug has been shown to have no anticholinergic activity. There is good evidence, however, that amantadine increases the release of both dopamine and norepinephrine in the peripheral and central nervous systems. It is similar in this regard to amphetamines but much less potent (Farnebo et al., 1971). The range of its therapeutic efficacy is similar to that of the anticholinergic compounds. The drug appears to be most effective when it is added to an existing treatment regimen consisting of anticholinergic agents or L-dopa or both (Yahr and DuVoisin, 1973).

Amphetamines

Of the drugs which have minor effects upon Parkinsonism, the amphetamines have the longest history. Dextroamphetamine (Dexedrine) is of mild benefit to patients with Parkinson's disease but its use for this purpose has been limited by its side effects and by the development of tolerance. The worst side effects are cardiovascular, particularly dangerous in the aged. More significant for our discussion, however, is the euphoria induced by amphetamines as well as the insomnia, loss of appetite, and occasional toxic psychosis which resembles schizophrenia very closely. Levoamphetamine has very little effect on mood, thought, appetite, or sleep and has not been used much in medical practice. Recent evidence indicates that it may, however, turn out to be quite beneficial for Parkinson's disease.

The amphetamines have been shown to increase the release of norepinephrine and inhibit its reuptake. D-amphetamine is about 10 times more potent than its L-isomer in inhibiting the reuptake-inactivation process of norepinephrine neurons in the brain, while the two isomers have similar potencies in dopamine neurons (Coyle and Snyder, 1969). Similarly, D-amphetamine is considerably more potent than L-amphetamine in releasing norepinephrine though these isomers have similar activities in effecting the release of dopamine (Taylor and Snyder, 1970). Thus, behavior which is mediated by norepinephrine should be affected much more by D- than by L-amphetamine, whereas behavior mediated by dopamine in the brain should be affected similarly by the two isomers of this drug. This prediction was substantiated in animal experiments that indicated a norepinephrine mediation of D-amphetamine-induced locomotor stimulation, whereas dopamine appeared to play the major role in the ability of amphetamine to elicit stereotyped compulsive behavior in rats (Taylor and Snyder, 1971).

This suggests that L-amphetamine might be at least as useful as D-amphetamine in Parkinson's disease and would be relatively free of the unpleasant side effects of D-amphetamine. If this hypothesis were substantiated it would also lend credence to the theory that central noradrenergic systems are more involved than dopaminergic systems in the mood, thought, appetite, and sleep changes induced by D-amphetamine. It could be taken as evidence that dopamine is more involved in the movement disorder than in the emotional and thought changes induced by D-amphetamine. This hypothesis has been incompletely tested in human beings but L-amphetamine appears to be quite effective in overcoming the drug-induced side effects in animals that resemble Parkinsonism (Snyder, 1970).

MAOI

Monamine oxidase inhibitors, especially tranylcypromine (Parnate) and isocarboxazid (Marplan) have proven useful in treating Parkinson's disease. These drugs probably produce their mild beneficial effect by partially alleviating the cerebral dopamine deficit. As overactivity of MAO is not a factor in the pathogenesis of Parkinsonism, the MAOI's would not be expected to have a major effect.

Tricyclics

The tricyclic antidepressants (imipramine and amitriptyline) are minimally effective in treating Parkinson's disease when used alone. In combination with other anti-Parkinsonian agents they may be very beneficial. These drugs act by inhibiting the uptake of norepinephrine and serotonin in peripheral and central neurons. (Himwich and Alpers, 1970). Their minor efficacy for the symptoms of Parkinson's disease may reflect the fact that they have very little effect on dopamine reuptake and may derive primarily from their antidepressant effect.

Parkinson-inducing Drugs
Reserpine and Phenothiazines

Reserpine and related natural and semisynthetic analogues are potent depleters of catecholamines and indoleamines because of their interference with the intraneuronal storage of amines. The marked depletion of norepinephrine, dopamine, and serotonin that reserpine causes is the basis for its clinical effects which are tranquilizing and antipsychotic, though the drug may induce Parkinsonism and/or depression. The other drugs that can induce Parkinsonism, the phenothiazines, butyrophenones, and thioxanthenes, have their primary biochemical action at the amine receptor sites where they competitively block receptors. Both dopamine and nor-epinephrine are synthesized at a faster rate after administration of these drugs. This can be interpreted as compensation for the blockade of catecholamine receptor sites. While the use of phenothiazines, butyrophenones and thioxanthenes is associated with an increase in the total brain-tissue level of catecholamines, the opposite of the res-erpine effect, these drugs share with reserpine the crucial action of re-ducing catecholamine concentration at the postsynaptic receptor site. Like reserpine, they are antipsychotic and tranquilizing but may exacerbate depression and induce Parkinsonism. Pronounced dystonia and other movement disorders are also side effects of these agents. If these movement disorders appear soon after medi-cation is started, they can virtually always be overcome by the in-jection of anticholinergic compounds. If phenothiazines must be administered on a long term basis, control of these drug-induced movement disorders can usually be maintained by the use of an anticholinergic compound. After months to years of treatment with these compounds, however, a form of movement disorder known as tardive dyskinesia can develop. This is a socially disabling disorder involving grimacing, chewing, and unsightly movements of the tongue and lips. It is also occasionally seen in older people who have not been taking any phenothiazine compounds. Discontinu-ing phenothiazines often does not help relieve the disorder, and administration of L-dopa and amantadine is usually ineffective (Ja-nowsky et al., 1972), though a few patients with tardive dyskinesia seem to benefit from the administration of amantadine. The bio-chemical aberration which presumably underlies the disorder has not yet been elucidated.

Alpha methylparatyrosine (α MPT) is a drug which inhibits tyrosine hydroxylase and thus brings the synthesis of both norepi-nephrine and dopamine to a halt. It has also been shown to induce Parkinsonism (Birkmayer, 1969) and ameliorate chorea (Chase, 1973) and the manic phase of manic-depressive illness (Bunney et al., 1971) and may potentiate the effect of phenothiazines in schizo-phrenia.

Intellectual and Emotional Changes in Parkinson Syndrome

In his original description of the syndrome, James Parkinson excluded intellectual change as one of the discriminating symptoms. In light of the clinical and biochemical similarity between Parkinsonism and depression (see p. 174), one might expect depressive symptoms to be more prominent in Parkinsonism patients. In this regard, Schwab et al. (1951) studied 200 patients who had Parkinson's disease for over five years. They noted four types of psychiatric complications in these patients: (1) Psychiatric disease unrelated to Parkinson's syndrome in that it existed before the onset of the Parkinsonian symptoms. (2) Reactive mental disorder brought on by disability. (3) Syndromes secondary to medication, especially psychotomimetic symptoms with anticholinergic drugs. (4) Paroxysmal disorders that he felt were specifically related to the Parkinsonian syndrome.

The paroxysmal disorders were most often noted in patients who also had oculogyric crises. These patients had anxiety attacks, even when there was no prior history or clear precipitating event. These anxiety attacks were terrifying to the patients, particularly when accompanied by feelings of imminent death. They were usually relieved by anti-Parkinsonian medication rather than by antianxiety agents. Schwab also described attacks of compulsive thinking, counting, and word use, depressive feelings, paranoid feelings, "strange feelings" in the limbs, and varied states of agitation, tension, and chronic fatigue. What was perhaps most noteworthy about these symptoms was their brevity and "attacklike" quality.

Mindham (1970) studied 89 patients with Parkinson's syndrome admitted to a psychiatric hospital and noted that 90 per cent of these patients showed depressive-mood disorder.

While it is clear there are mood changes in Parkinson's syndrome, it is unclear if there are intellectual changes. Garon et al. (1972) found that patients with marked akinesia beginning late in life suffered more intellectual deterioration than a group with less pronounced akinesia and earlier onset. Donelly and Chase (1973) did not confirm the finding of intellectual deterioration but noted that after L-dopa treatment, full-scale I.Q. and memory function as measured by the WAIS increased. The improvement was evident both at one month and seventeen months after the initiation of treatment. They found no relation of intellectual dysfunction and any motor difficulty.

In dealing with supposed mental changes in Parkinsonian patients, one of the major problems is that the etiology of the syndrome varies and some of the diseases which cause Parkinsonism, such as arteriosclerosis, also cause dementia. Another problem is that the older patient with Parkinsonism is likely to be senile or to have suffered intellectual deterioration caused by some process entirely independent of that causing Parkinsonism.

Riklan and Levita (1969) have had the opportunity to study a large group of patients subjected to neurosurgical ablations of various portions of the extrapyramidal tract for movement disorders. The patients who showed the greatest intellectual changes after destruction of these areas were those who had bilateral rather than unilateral operations. In the immediate postoperative period there was a general decline in intellectual functioning, diminished drive and productivity, and loss of perceptual motor integration. Patients with ablations in the left hemisphere showed greater loss of verbal functioning than those with ablations in the right hemisphere. The right-hemisphere group showed more changes in emotional reactivity. At six month follow-up, however, all the patients seemed to return to their preoperative level of functioning. The patients with bilateral lesions, however, not only took longer to recover at follow-up but seemed to show decreases in initiative and motivation.

CHOREA

Clinical Features and Physiologic Considerations

Chorea consists of involuntary jerky movements of the face, tongue, extremities, especially the distal portions and even the trunk and respiratory muscles in some patients. Choreatic movements are rapid and irregular and they become more pronounced during voluntary movement and attempts to maintain a posture. Patients with chorea tend to "cover up" their disability by blending the pseudopurposeful choreatic movements with normal voluntary movements. Sometimes while walking a patient may show a slight lilt to his gait and will appear to be dancing. Choreatic movements can sometimes be revealed by having a patient squeeze the examiner's fingers. The choreatic movements of the patient's fingers which this accentuates gives the examiner the sensation of being milked, hence the term "milkmaid's sign." Patients with chorea are often unable to maintain protrusion of the tongue, and when they put their arms above their heads choreatic movements of the upper extremities are maximized and the hands tend to pronate (pronator's sign). Choreatic movements superimposed upon deep tendon reflexes cause the relaxation phase of the reflex to be discontinuous (hung-up reflexes).

Chorea and the slower writhing movements of athetosis (with which it is often associated and from which it cannot always be clearly distinguished) may be manifestations of one of several diseases: perinatal brain injury, encephalitis, vascular disease, hypoparathyroidism, Wilson's disease, and, rarely, brain tumor.

Huntington's chorea is a degenerative disease of the brain involving the cortical mantle as well as the basal ganglia. Because of the prominent involvement of the caudate nucleus and putamen in this disease, it has been suggested that chorea may be related to pathology of the striatum. It would, however, be a mistake to identify chorea with pathology of the striatum solely, because of the extensive striatal connections to the caudate, globus pallidus, and thalamus. Chorea may be the result of an interruption of or imbalance between other neural systems, e.g., inhibitory and excitatory motor pathways, in the striatal-pallidal-thalamic circuit. Carrea and Mettler (1955) produced transitory choreatic activity in monkeys by placing bilateral lesions in the superior cerebellar peduncles.

Unilateral lesions of the ventral-lateral thalamus and subthalamic nuclei in man and in monkeys sometimes produce choreatic movements. Chorea in such cases is hypothesized as resulting from the loss of inhibiting influences on the globus pallidus. Virtually all the diseases in which chorea occurs may be associated with severe emotional disturbance. Roughly half of the patients with Huntington's chorea present themselves with psychiatric symptoms and half develop psychosis at some point in the illness. Twenty-five per cent of these are indistinguishable from schizophrenia (Heathfield, 1967). Emotional disturbances frequently accompany Sydenham's chorea and may persist for many years (Freeman et al., 1965). Psychosis and signs of dementia may be prominent in Wilson's disease; and in encephalitis, of course, emotional changes are common. All of the conditions that cause chorea involve the brain diffusely, and emotional changes are not always present. These changes derive from involvement of parts of the nervous system that have little or no relation to those which give rise to chorea. Psychosis is thus a frequent, though not an obligatory, concomitant of chorea.

Effect of Medications

The drugs that help to alleviate chorea are those which can induce Parkinsonism, i.e., reserpine, phenothiazines, and the other major tranquilizers, and α methyl paratyrosine (α MPT). As mentioned above, all these drugs reduce catecholamine concentrations at their receptor sites; reserpine by depleting catecholamine from the nervous system entirely, phenothiazines and related compounds by competitively blocking catecholamine at receptor sites, and α MPT by blocking catecholamine synthesis.

Drugs which potentiate catecholamine activity worsen chorea. These include belladonna compounds (Aquilonius and Sjöström, 1971; Klawans, and Rubovits, 1972;) and imipramine (Whittier, 1961). Of the drugs that worsen chorea, L-dopa is by far the most prominent. About half of all people receiving L-dopa in therapeutic doses for Parkinson's disease develop a choreatic movement disorder. L-dopa has been shown to worsen the movement disorder in patients with Huntington's chorea and this has led to the suggestion that it might be useful in the detection of presymptomatic Huntington's chorea. Klawans and co-workers (1972) gave low to moderate doses of L-dopa to the asymptomatic offspring of patients with Huntington's chorea. Roughly one-third developed chorea and it was assumed that these individuals were carriers of a gene for the disease and would develop it in time. Follow-up studies have not yet been done.

Although the effects of amphetamines upon chorea have not been systematically studied, patients who have taken overdoses of amphetamines either acutely or chronically may develop symptoms of restlessness, tremor, motor impersistence, and "jumpiness" which strongly resemble choreiform movements. Motor signs of amphetamine overdosage are minor in comparison with the abnormal mental state produced by amphetamine intoxication, however.

Since chorea is improved by drugs which have an antidopaminergic effect and worsened or induced by drugs which augment dopamine activity it has been hypothesized that chorea is the result of excessive dopaminergic activity or sensitivity. The pharmacologic evidence which suggests that the extrapyramidal signs and symptoms of Huntington's chorea may be related to a hypersensitivity of dopamine receptors in the striatum to endogenous dopamine has been summarized by Klawans (1970). When the brains of patients with Huntington's chorea are examined at autopsy, the basal ganglia, especially the caudate and putamen are characteristically depleted of neurons. Despite the severe loss of neurons, the dopamine content of the putamen and globus pallidus per gram of remaining tissue has been found to be normal and that of the caudate reduced to approximately 60 per cent of normal. Since the number of neurons per gram is greatly reduced in Huntington's chorea in these regions, it has been hypothesized that each striatal neuron remaining in this disease may contain or be exposed to a relative excess of dopamine. Alternatively, it has been suggested that a change of dopaminergic balance in the basal ganglia occurs, favoring pallidum and putamen over the caudate, and that a relative dopaminergic excess in the putamen-pallidum system causes chorea (Bernheimer and Hornykiewicz, 1973). In summary, there is pharmacologic and some biochemical evidence that chorea results from excess dopamine or excessive sensitivity to dopamine. According to this view, chorea is pathophysiologically and biochemically the opposite of Parkinsonism (Klawans, 1970).

DEPRESSION

The fact that many drugs and neurotransmitters that improve or worsen Parkinson's syndrome are also effective in treating or inducing depression suggests that the two disorders may have a similar biochemical background. While this is an inadequate basis for conclusions about the etiology of depression, the clinical and pharmacological evidence strongly implies the existence of biochemical disturbance in affective disorders. In recent years, research has been more fruitful in elucidating the biochemical aspects of depression than of any other psychiatric disorder.

Clinical Features and Nosology

The major phenomenology of affective illness (depression or mania) is mood disturbance. Depressed feelings are usually described as sadness, feeling "blue," "low," or gloomy. Because of the ubiquity of these feelings, it is not clear when to consider them pathological. Usually, this judgment is made on clinical grounds by weighing such factors as the severity of the symptoms, the amount of interference they cause with the functioning of the individual, the duration of the symptoms, the age at which they occur, the number of similar episodes previously experienced by the patient, and the presence of a family history of similar disturbances. Because quantitation of these factors is so difficult, diagnostic confusion often occurs and this has resulted in an impressive diversity of classifications used for depressive disorders. In the literature one finds such adjectives for depression as psychotic, neurotic, endogenous, reactive, agitated, retarded, involutional, and postpartum. These distinctions are descriptive deriving primarily from the etiologic theory the author espouses.

Most classifications that impute etiologic differences to different states of depression must be tentative in our present state of knowledge (Blumer et al., 1971). Even the common distinction between reactive (psychologic) and endogenous (biologic) depression seems arbitrary, for every depressive state must have both a psychologic and biologic component. Findings that usually lead to the classification of depression as reactive are: the presence of precipitating factors, a history of previous neurotic traits, good insight, early night sleep disturbance, and emotional lability. The factors invoked to support the diagnosis of endogenous depression are: delusions, psychomotor retardation, diurnal variation, and a family history of depression. This distinction between reactive and endogenous depression creates some problems. (1) The significance of a particular life event to which an individual is supposed to be reacting is determined only after he becomes depressed. Thus, the causal relationship between the depression and the event presumed to have caused it is a matter of post hoc reasoning. It is seldom possible to predict whether an individual will become significantly depressed after a particular event. As depressed patients frequently either distort life events or overemphasize their unfavorable side, these allegedly causal events may actually be a product of the depressive feelings themselves. (2) The diversity in individuals' reactions to events that might be expected to evoke depression indicates that pre-existing constitutional factors determine the timing and severity of "reactive" depression and these constitutional factors are, of course, endogenous. (3) The use of the terms reactive and endogenous by clinicians frequently depends more on the severity of the symptoms than on the precipitating factors. If a patient's symptomatology is only moderate, not psychotic, and his functioning is not markedly impaired, the clinician frequently and arbitrarily will classify the depression as reactive. The severity of illness is not always a logical basis for this distinction because many patients suffering episodes of psychotic depression also experience episodes of milder depression and both the mild and severe forms respond to antidepressant medications. Consequently, it is not likely that the distinction between "reactive" and "endogenous" depressions reflects a different biochemical pathogenesis. They are not necessarily different conditions, but different points on a spectrum of severity. Kendall (1968) has shown in longitudinal and cross-sectional studies of depressed patients that use of the labels "reactive" and "endogenous" or "neurotic" and "psychotic" often emphasizes the extremes of a symptomatic continuum and ignores the middle ground.

There are three types of depressive symptoms: (1) disturbance of mood; (2) alteration in the person's perception of himself and the environment surrounding him; and (3) biological disturbances. Patients with altered mood are aware that their mood has changed. In moderate or severe depressions patients perceive themselves as being worthless, hopeless, helpless, guilty, even at times "evil." Frequently they view their accomplishments as meaningless and neither persuasion nor confrontation with reality can change their attitude. If they are delusional the delusions usually relate to ideas of bodily illness, decay, or other dismal eventualities. In manic conditions we see the obverse of these feelings: euphoria, grandiosity, and a heightened sense of one's abilities. Among the body functions that may be disrupted are sleep, appetite, digestion, sexual activity, and psychomotor activity. Sleep disturbances are often manifested as hyposomnia, difficulty in falling asleep, awakening frequently throughout the night, early morning awakening, or any combination of these. Many depressed patients sleep excessively (hypersomnia). Anorexia, weight loss, or hyperphagia, and weight gain are common. Decreased sexual interest and activity are the rule.

Changes in psychomotor function, either agitation or retardation, are frequently evident. Agitated patients seem anxious, wring their hands, pace about, and frequently sleep poorly. Psychomotor retardation is characterized by reduced physical and mental activity and often by hypersomnia. The slowing of thought processes in retarded depressions may suggest dementia. Suicidal ideation is usually prominent in severe depression.

If the symptoms of depression are *present in mild form and transiently* (not lasting more than six months) and follow emotionally charged events (usually loss of job, health, or a loved one), the reaction may be considered as grief (Parkes, 1970). If the symptoms are severe, regardless of the presence of precipitants, if they persist, and if they interfere with the patient's functioning from day to day, the condition should be regarded as depressive illness and should be treated. The severity of a depressive syndrome is best characterized by summing up the symptoms rather than weighing individual symptoms differently. Recently, scales for quantitating the severity and variety of affective symptoms have been devised (Hamilton, 1969; Beck et al., 1971 and Zung, 1965). We have found such phenomenological classification to be quite useful. It is a relatively reliable method of judging the severity of depression, following the course of the disorder, and evaluating therapy.

The duration and tendency of depression to recur as well as the severity of symptoms vary from patient to patient. In some patients depression occurs as a single episode in an otherwise normal life. Most patients having their first depression have no family history of depression. When the family history is negative, there is no way of predicting the course of illness. The chances are that a remission will occur and that the symptoms will respond to antidepressant medication. There is probably a greater likelihood that such a patient will again become depressed in the future than someone of the same age and sex who has never been clinically depressed, but information on this point is sketchy.

Other patients have repeated episodes of affective disorder and their illnesses may be divided into two groups:

(a) Unipolar—manifested by repeated depressive (or rarely manic) episodes.

(b) Bipolar—characterized by repeated episodes of both mania and depression. In some bipolar patients mania is more prevalent, almost to the exclusion of depression, and the opposite may occur. In such cases, the diagnosis of bipolarity rests upon other clinical characteristics and genetic data. Family studies indicate that while both unipolar and bipolar depressions are familial, there is no genetic overlap between the two; that is, bipolar illness does not occur in the families of monopolar probands and vice versa. The parents and siblings of bipolar patients have a 20 per cent risk of bipolar illness and the parents and siblings of unipolar patients (defined in these studies as patients with more than three episodes of depression) have a 12 to 14 per cent risk of unipolar depressive disease (Slater and Cowie, 1971).

The mode by which recurrent depressive disorders are inherited is not clear, but the fact that they are inherited is virtually indisputable. Twin studies of the affective disorders have been limited to bipolar illness which affects less than one per cent of the general population. A review of these studies indicates the all-over concordance rate for bipolar disease to be 72 per cent in monozygotic pairs and 19 per cent in same-sexed dizygotic pairs (not age corrected). In Kallman's series, concordance rates for monozygotic pairs reached 96 per cent.

Other differences distinguish unipolar and bipolar depression. The sex ratio in bipolar illness is one to one but unipolar depression is twice as common in females as in males. Color blindness and the Xg blood group have been linked with bipolar but not unipolar illness (Winokur et al., 1971). The average age at the time of occurrence of the first episode of unipolar depression severe enough to require hospitalization is forty-five; bipolar depressions of such severity first occur on the average at age thirty (Detre and Jarecki,

1971). In a review of follow-up studies of unipolar and bipolar affective disorders, Robins and Guze (1972) noted that the median duration of the first attack of a depressive illness varied. In unipolar depression it was 13 months, in bipolar depressions it was 6.5 months. The mean duration of manic attacks was 3.5 months. Individual unipolar depressions last longer than bipolar ones but they are less likely to relapse. Between episodes of illness, unipolar patients tend to be insecure, sensitive, or obsessional while bipolar patients tend to be more active and sociable. Biegel and Murphy (1971) compared the clinical characteristics of the depressive state in 25 patients diagnosed as having bipolar illness and in 25 patients with unipolar depressive illness. Patients were observed for a 14-day drug-free period in a research ward during which time mania was absent. Greater physical activity, more overt expressions of anger, and more somatic complaints distinguished the unipolar from the bipolar patients, who tended to be less active and more socially withdrawn. The difference had statistical significance. Some authors have emphasized the tendency of unipolar depressions to be agitated with hyposomnia and bipolar depressions to be retarded with hypersomnia (Detre et al., 1972).

In summary, we believe that depression falls into the following general categories: (1) grief reactions, (2) nonrecurrent depression which may or may not occur in relation to environmental stresses, and may or may not be inherited, and (3) recurrent affective disorder, either bipolar (manic-depressive) or unipolar.

Biologic Changes in Depression

It is often difficult to interpret biologic studies of depression because of the varied diagnostic categories. Only recently have such clear phenomenological distinctions as unipolar and bipolar depression been made. Therefore, earlier studies and those lacking clear, clinical descriptions must be interpreted with caution. It is noteworthy, however, that the soft signs of diffuse neurologic dysfunction and the EEG abnormalities so often present in schizophrenic patients are not found in many studies of depressed patients. There is little or no EEG change in bipolar patients when they go from depression to mania or vice versa.

Sacher (1967) found that depressed patients have elevated blood and urine levels of corticosteroids. While this may be a secondary effect related to the stress of a depressive illness, it is noteworthy that elevated steroid levels may affect the metabolism of biogenic amines (Curzon, 1971). Coppen (1967) has documented increased total body sodium and specifically increased intracellular sodium concentration in both depressed and manic states. It has also been shown that lithium, which is interchangeable with sodium, decreases the intracellular exchange of sodium and normalizes the cortico-steroid disturbance. This may have something to do with the effect of lithium in alleviating mania and depression. In depressed states it has been shown that there is in general diminished secretion of gastric juice and saliva, reduced peristalsis, and a decreased basal metabolic rate.

Hypothalamic dysfunction in depression is suggested by sleep disturbances, slowed heart rate, lowered body temperature, loss of weight and appetite, disturbances of the menstrual cycle, and impotence and frigidity (Hill, 1968; Pollitt, 1965). A general state of hyperarousal has been demonstrated in the depressed patient. Some studies (Whatmore and Ellis, 1962) in depressed patients have shown both elevated galvanic skin responses and muscle tension (Whybrow and Mendels, 1969). Buchsbaum and colleagues (1971) noted a tendency in depressed patients to augment the intensity of incoming stimuli.

Sleep disturbance is one of the most consistent features of depressive illness. In general, it parallels depression in severity. Conventional wisdom in the past, supported mainly by clinical impressions, identified early morning awakening with depressive psychosis (Noyes and Kolb, 1963), involutional melancholia (English and Finch, 1954), and endogenous depression (Kiloh and Garside, 1963) as opposed to neurotic or reactive depression in which difficulty falling asleep was supposed to be characteristic. In more recent quantitative EEG-controlled studies, the clinical impression of early morning awakening as a distinguishing feature of these "different types" of depression was not borne out (Hawkins and Mendels, 1966), though hyposomnia was found to be a characteristic of most depressive illness. This is manifested as early-morning wakefulness, a longer latency of sleep onset, and a decrease in non-rapid eye movement sleep, both absolute and relative to total sleep. In contrast to other forms of depressive illness, the depressive phase of bipolar depressive illness is often characterized by increased total sleep and increased relative and total time spent in the rapid-eye-movement (REM) stage of sleep. During the manic phase, total sleep time is always lower as is the percentage in the REM phase (E. Hartman, 1968; Detre et al., 1972).

In summary, then, depressed patients commonly undergo a decrease in many physiological functions in their responsiveness to a wide range of stimuli. This is accompanied by a heightened state of arousal which may be experienced by the patient as anxiety or tension. These alterations of normal function can be corrected by modern therapy, and the most interesting correlation between the resumption of normal behavioral and biological function is provided by the use of antidepressant drugs.

Treatment

In evaluating the treatment of depression there are two prevailing difficulties: the above-mentioned absence of a definitive classification of depression, and the fact that even chronic, recurrent depressive illnesses usually have time-limited episodes. Nevertheless, the therapeutic efficacy of the tricyclic antidepressants (imipramine and amitriptyline) is well substantiated. Sixty to seventy per cent of depressed patients benefit from the use of these drugs (Kuhn, 1958; Klein and David, 1969; Greenblatt et al., 1964), whether they are older patients with "endogenous" psychotic depressions or young patients with "reactive" depressions (Witten-born et al., 1962; Abraham et al., 1963).

The major untoward reactions associated with the use of tricyclic antidepressants (dry mouth, blurred vision, and urinary retention) can be attributed to their anticholinergiclike effect. Occasionally, a full blown encephalopathy with thought disorder and seizures has been reported (Davies et al., 1971). Imipramine, though some-times helpful in relieving the rigidity of patients with Parkinson's disease, has been known to aggravate the tremor. Imipramine has also been reported to aggravate chorea in depressed patients with Huntington's chorea (Whittier et al., 1961).

The tricyclic antidepressants are generally thought to exert their effects through inhibition of norepinephrine reuptake in the pe-ripheral and central noradrenergic neurons. Recently, however, it has been demonstrated that the reuptake of serotonin can also be blocked by the tricyclic antidepressants (Sulser and Sanders-Bush, 1971). The question arises whether the clinical antidepressant ac-tivity of this class of drugs is more closely related to their effects on serotonin or norepinephrine neurons. At present, it appears that tri-cyclic inhibition of norepinephrine reuptake may produce their ef-fect on psychomotor activity while their inhibition of serotonin reuptake may be responsible for the brightening of mood in de-pressed patients (Carlsson et al., 1969). It is also conceivable that the therapeutic response depends on the relationship between nor-epinephrine and serotonin content of the brain (Schildkraut, 1973).

The monamine oxidase inhibitors produce almost all of the side effects reported for the tricyclics, including confusional syndromes. The MAOI's do not have as broad a range of antidepressant effects as the tricyclics, and it is not entirely clear that their antidepressant action is the result of inhibition of monamine oxidase since these drugs have many other effects on neural metabolism. Hypertensive crises that follow consumption of certain tryptamine-containing foods in patients receiving the MAOI's most certainly do relate to their inhibition of monamine oxidase, however.

There is general agreement that episodes of mania can be brought to an end within 10 days by the administration of lithium carbonate and that chronic lithium therapy prevents the recurrence of manic episodes in most individuals suffering from bipolar disease. Eighty per cent of manic patients show distinct improvement after the initial lag period. The more certain the diagnosis of mania, the more likely the therapeutic response (Davis et al., 1973). Recent longitudinal studies of a large group of manic-depressive patients (Baastrup and Schou, 1967) showed that the average relapse rate was once every eight months. After institution of lithium treatment the relapse rate dropped to once every sixty months. When lithium treatment was stopped, almost all of the patients had relapses within three to four months (Baastrup and Schou, 1967). Studies by Angst et al. (1970), Small et al. (1971), and a carefully controlled double blind study by Baastrup et al. (1970) all confirmed the above findings, indicating that lithium is an effective prophylactic in preventing relapses of either manic or depressive nature.

The use of lithium in treating schizoaffective disorders and other periodic behavioral disturbances is under investigation but preliminary results indicate that it is much less effective for them than for mania. While the mechanism of action of lithium is not yet established for certain, there are some indications that it accelerates presynaptic catabolism of norepinephrine, inhibits the release of norepinephrine and serotonin, and stimulates the norepinephrine uptake process (Davis and Fann, 1971).

Murphy and coworkers (1971) have shown that L-dopa in therapeutic doses can regularly induce manic episodes in some bipolar patients. Patients with unipolar depression fail to benefit from the use of L-dopa but do not develop mania while taking the drug. When depressed patients are divided into retarded and agitated groups, the retarded group seems to benefit somewhat from L-dopa. Agitated depression, if anything, tends to become worse (Murphy et al., 1971).

As mentioned above, the amphetamines have an euphoric effect upon individuals who take them in large doses. At one time the amphetamines were the only drugs used for depression. They were not especially effective in treating depression, and their use had to be curtailed because of side effects and development of tolerance. With the spread of drug abuse, many physicians have become acquainted with the effects of amphetamine overdose and withdrawal.

Amphetamines, as we have already mentioned, are known to have several biochemical effects. They reduce the reuptake of norepinephrine and facilitate its release. There is some evidence that d-amphetamine has a direct effect upon noradrenergic receptors. Both these effects potentiate the action of norepinephrine. The drugs also may inhibit tyrosine hydroxylase activity and by so doing reduce the synthesis of both dopamine and norepinephrine. With continued use, amphetamines lead to a depletion of norepinephrine in the nervous system. This could explain the tolerance which develops with chronic use of d-amphetamine (Cooper et al., 1971).

When amphetamine is withdrawn there should presumably be a lag before depleted catecholamine stores return to normal. This lag period would correspond to the depression ("crash") which is regularly seen in dexedrine-users who have suddenly stopped taking the drug.

Amine Hypothesis

The results of these clinical trials have led to the catecholamine hypothesis of depression (Schildkraut, 1970). According to this theory a certain level of amines and of receptor sensitivity to these neurotransmitters is necessary for normal mood. If the amine receptors are insensitive or if there is a deficiency in amine synthesis, storage, release, or ability to reach the receptor, there will be depression. If the receptors are hypersensitive, or if there is an excess of active amines, mania and/or psychosis will develop. The results of

the drug studies reviewed above are consistent with this interpretation.

The MAOI's and tricyclic inhibitors improve depression and
worsen or induce mania. They also increase catcholamine concentration at postsynaptic receptors. The same is true of amphetamines. Although L-dopa, the catecholamine precursor, does not
primarily relieve depression, high doses may induce mania. There
is some question as to whether belladonna compounds relieve depression through their inhibiting effect on the reuptake process.
Conversely, reserpine and the phenothiazines, which reduce the
amount of transmitter available at the dendritic receptor sites, induce or increase depression and are occasionally effective in treating mania. Lithium, which is effective in blocking episodes of mania may act by decreasing release, and increasing reuptake and
catabolism of norepinephrine and thus may have exactly the opposite effect from that of tricyclic mood elevators. There is not as
yet enough information available to explain how lithium might act
prophylactically to prevent recurrent bipolar depressions.

Recently, Janowsky and coworkers (1971) demonstrated that
manic symptoms could be suppressed, at least transiently, by administration of an acetylcholinesterase inhibitor, physostigmine.
The suppression occurred only with physostigmine and not with
a placebo or a noncentrally acting cholinesterase inhibitor, neostig-
mine. They hypothesized that mania may be a disease of "relative
adrenergic predominance" and depression a disease of "relative cholinergic predominance." They also noted that schizophrenic and
manic patients receiving methylphenidate manifested increased
talkativeness and activity and that this effect was antagonized by
physostigmine. This is an interesting theory as it raises the possibility that the biochemical basis of both mania and depression are related to the proper balance of neurotransmitters rather than to
merely a deficiency of any single substance. The conceptualization of depression as a state of inhibition and mania as a state of
activation is consistent with the physiological findings of CNS hy-

perexcitability in both mania and depression. Mania would reflect this hyperexcitability when it "breaks through" the state of inhibition, depression.

This is really the same "balance" theory of cholinergic and adrenergic mechanisms which has been put forward to explain movement disorders. Physostigmine worsens Parkinsonism and reduces chorea. The mechanism by which these changes are produced is assumed to be the result of its antiacetylcholinesterase activity but it has not yet been determined if physostigmine has a direct action upon brain amines.

PSYCHOSIS

The symptoms of psychosis, or thought disorder, have been discussed in Chapter 3, along with some of the clinical considerations by means of which one can distinguish idiopathic (familial) schizophrenia from the schizophrenialike psychosis of epilepsy and the psychoses associated with neurological diseases and drug effects. The similarities between drug-induced psychosis and schizophrenia are, on balance, more striking than the differences and this has been the basis for several speculations about the etiology of psychosis.

For many years it has been known that mescaline and amphetamines can induce psychosis. The structural similarity between these methylated compounds and the catecholamines (*Fig.* 5-2) prompted the suggestion that abnormal methylation of catecholamines may lead to the formation of an amine with psychotogenic properties. The search for such an amine in schizophrenics has led into many blind alleys. One of the most promising findings was the discovery by Friedhoff and Van Winkle (1962) of 3,4 dimethoxyphenylethylamine (DMPEA) in the urine of schizophrenic patients. This is a nonpsychotogenic dimethylated derivative of dopamine, identical to mescaline except that it lacks one methoxy group. It was thought possible that DMPEA might be a metabolite of a psychotogenic precursor in schizophrenic patients. As it turned out, excretion of this compound is influenced by both drugs and diet, especially

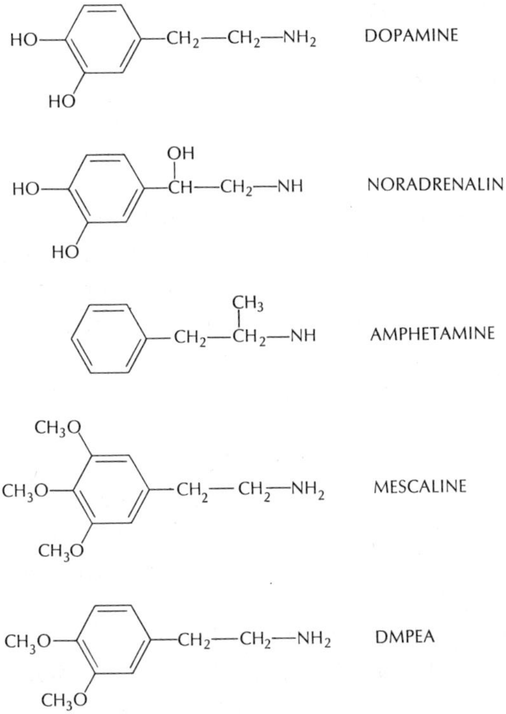

FIG. 5-2
STRUCTURE OF SOME
AMINES

those to which institutionalized psychiatric patients are exposed. It can also be found in the urine of some normal individuals.

Another approach to investigating the possibility that an abnormally methylated amine could cause schizophrenia was the infusion of methyl donors (methionine and betaine) into schizophrenics, other psychiatric patients and normal individuals (Kety, 1967). While toxic to some degree to all groups, these compounds clearly worsened the schizophrenic symptoms of schizophrenic patients. This rather frail reed is the only present support for the theory that abnormally methylated compounds cause schizophrenia.

Though there is no direct evidence that in schizophrenia either an abnormal amine or an excess of normal amine exists, drugs that affect amines can produce, worsen, or alleviate schizophrenia or schizophrenialike psychoses. In discussing these drugs we will limit ourselves to the agents already mentioned in the sections on the movement and affective disorders.

The first effective antipsychotic drugs were the rauwolfia alkaloids, of which reserpine was the most widely used. They have proven to be effective in reducing impulsivity, agitation, excitement and chronic paranoid irritability. Such side effects as hypotension, gastrointestinal bleeding, impotence, and depression, together with the long half-life of the compounds which makes control of side effects by dosage adjustment difficult, have led most psychiatrists to prefer phenothiazines and related major tranquilizers for the treatment of psychosis. The phenothiazines are especially helpful in controlling the following symptoms of psychosis: psychomotor agitation, delusional and paranoid ideation, auditory hallucinations, blocking, inappropriate affect, and social withdrawal (Goldberg et al., 1965). The phenothiazines are as effective in treating drug-induced psychosis as in idiopathic schizophrenia. The antipsychotic effects of rauwolfia alkaloids and phenothiazines could be understood if psychosis were shown to result from abnormal amines, an excess of normal catecholamines or indoleamines, or receptor hypersensitivity to normal amines.

The same hypothesis can be invoked to explain the effect of drugs known to worsen or induce psychosis whose mechanisms of action have already been discussed. The amphetamines, chronic use of which leads to a psychotic state virtually indistinguishable from paranoid schizophrenia, potentiates release of amines. Amphetamines also may be active themselves at amine receptor sites. Anticholinergics and tricyclic mood elevators which reduce amine uptake may induce psychosis in some sensitive, nonpsychotic individuals and may cause worsening of psychosis in schizophrenics. Amantadine which can induce a drug psychosis, acts by enhancing amine release. The MAOI's which prevent the degradative metabolism of both catechol- and indoleamines can worsen or induce psychosis in sensitive individuals. L-dopa which is a precursor of both dopamine and norepinephrine causes confusion, paranoia, agitation, and excitement in roughly 5 per cent of patients receiving it for Parkinsonism and tends to aggravate pre-existing psychotic problems (Yaryura-Tobias et al., 1970).

SLEEP

Before leaving the subject of biogenic amines and brain disorders, it seems appropriate to review some of the salient features of narcolepsy. If we could understand this condition, we would have taken a great step in bridging the hiatus between psychosis and neurochemistry; for narcolepsy features a sleep disturbance, motor alterations, hallucinations, EEG changes, and is remarkably affected by drugs which influence cerebral amines.

Narcolepsy consists of four cardinal symptoms: sleep attacks, cataplexy, sleep paralysis, and hypnagogic hallucinations. In only 10 per cent of cases in which the diagnosis is made are all four symptoms present. In 70 per cent of cases, sleep attacks and cataplexy exist alone. There is often a family history of narcolepsy which spans several generations. This has led to the proposal of a single, dominant mode of inheritance (Zarcone, 1973).

The SLEEP ATTACKS may be sudden, coming on without warning, or they may be preceded by an irresistible urge to sleep. The attacks vary in duration, lasting from several minutes to an hour or more. In some cases, patients are normally alert between attacks but others are constantly drowsy and become drowsier as they tire, especially toward the end of the working day. These patients often fall asleep under boring social circumstances conducive to sleep. This is often misunderstood and patients are considered lazy, impolite, neurotic, or worse. The most serious threat posed by the condition is accidental death which results from a sleep attack or cataplectic attack. Automobile accidents are a much more frequent complication of narcolepsy than of epilepsy. Forty per cent of narcoleptics admitted that they had fallen asleep while driving (Bartels and Kuskacioglu, 1965).

CATAPLEXY can be defined as the sudden loss of muscle tone that causes a patient to slump or fall to the floor. It is unassociated with unconsciousness and it is usually precipitated by a strong, sudden emotion such as laughter, anger, or surprise. It is usually brief, lasting several seconds to several minutes.

The first two symptoms are the most incapacitating and are more likely to cause a patient to seek medical attention than the remaining two. SLEEP PARALYSIS is a state which occurs on awakening and affects all skeletal muscles except those of respiration and the extraocular muscles (EOM). It typically lasts for a few seconds to a few minutes and is associated with alertness, a desire to get up, great fear, and often with vivid visual and auditory nightmares which persist from the sleeping into the waking states and are called *hypnagogic hallucinations.*

The entire narcolepsy syndrome was once considered to be purely "functional" as it was unassociated with any objective abnormality; the EEG in the waking state is normal. Sophisticated psychological explanations for the phenomena were provided by some on a post hoc basis. The condition thus serves as a reminder that our classification of disease as functional is more often a reflection of our ignorance than our cleverness.

Sleep studies of the last decade have indicated that sleep can be divided into several stages, perhaps the most important being the REM (rapid eye movement) and non-REM phases. The former is associated with a desynchronized EEG, with loss of muscle tone in all skeletal muscles except the EOM and muscles of respiration, and with dreaming. The non-REM phase is associated with high voltage slow wave electroencephalographic activity and normal skeletal muscle tone. Dreaming does not occur in this phase. In normal controls, REM phases occur in intervals of ever increasing duration beginning about 90 minutes after the onset of sleep and ultimately account for about 20 per cent of total sleeping time. Patients with narcolepsy, however, characteristically enter the REM phase immediately after falling asleep and spend more time in REM sleep than do controls (Dement et al., 1966).

Narcolepsy is now considered to be the result of overactivity of the REM system: sleep attacks are episodic REM sleep phases; cataplexy and sleep paralysis are the result of REM-associated loss of muscle tone which spares only the EOM and respiratory muscles; hypnagogic hallucinations are persistent REM-associated dreams.

The ideal drug for the treatment of narcolepsy would have the effect of reducing REM attacks without increasing non-REM sleep or producing drowsiness. Virtually all sedatives reduce REM but clearly they could not be used to treat narcolepsy. Amphetamines in large doses at present are the drugs of choice, though they only ameliorate sleep attacks and do not affect the other symptoms of narcolepsy. All the side effects which attend their use in other conditions are encountered in narcolepsy and amphetamines may well be the cause of the high incidence of "schizophrenia" in narcolepsy (Sours, 1963).

Other drugs which potentiate amine action and reduce REM may be effective in narcolepsy. MAO inhibitors relieve all four of the symptoms even in previously intractable cases (Wyatt et al., 1971), and imipramine is effective in relieving cataplexy (Hishikowa et al., 1966). Other drugs discussed in this chapter have not been systematically investigated in relation to narcolepsy.

Several observations suggest that brain serotonin is intimately involved in the biochemistry of sleep. Non-REM sleep is potentiated and REM sleep suppressed by parenteral injections of the serotonin precursor 5-hydroxytroptophane or by intraventricular injection of serotonin. Non-REM sleep is reduced when brain serotonin is reduced by blocking its synthesis with p-chlorophenylalanine.

Reserpine also reduces non-REM sleep and triggers the EEG components of REM sleep (Jouvet, 1969).

REM sleep has also been thought to be dependent upon a cholinergic mechanism because it is suppressed by atropine. In view of the evidence that synthetic atropinelike drugs inhibit catecholamine uptake (Coyle and Snyder, 1969), it may be that atropine suppresses REM and potentiates non-REM sleep by this mechanism which is shared by the tricyclic antidepressants.

Sleep disorders are common concomitants of anxiety, affective disorders, and schizophrenia. Most movement disorders stop during sleep. Investigations concerning the role of biogenic amines in producing the sleep disturbances seen in these psychiatric conditions and the relationship of neurological diseases to sleep has only just started.

SUMMARY

It may be worthwhile to summarize the data and hypotheses presented in this chapter even at the risk of further oversimplifying a complicated subject. There is a good deal of evidence that disturbances in dopaminergic functions are the biochemical basis of both Parkinson's disease and chorea. In the former, there is a lack of dopamine and in the latter a relative excess. There is some clinical similarity between Parkinsonism and depression and features of depression are seen in Parkinson's disease. According to the catecholamine hypothesis of depression, a decrease in catecholamine (mainly norepinephrine) and serotonin activity causes depression and an excess causes mania. This theory derives mainly from what is known about the mechanism of action of drugs that relieve or induce depression. The evidence supporting the theory is thus indirect. The kind of evidence that supports the catecholamine hypothesis of depression suggests that thought disorders are related to excessive reactivity to amines whether catecholamines, indoleamines, or other biogenic amines or some combination thereof.

Table 5-1
Catecholamines
Drugs, Movement, Mood, and Psychosis

Drugs	Parkinson's	Depression	Mania	Psychosis	Chorea	Probable Major Amine Mechanism
Anticholinergics	better	?better	?	worse	worse	Inhibits DA Uptake
L-dopa	better	?better	worse	worse	worse	↑ DA synthesis
Phenothiazines	worse	worse	better	better	better	Blocks postsynaptic receptors of DA & NE
MAO inhibitors	better	better	worse	worse	worse	↓ catabolism of DA, NE, and serotonin in presynaptic cell
Imipramine	?better	better	worse	worse	worse	Inhibits NE and serotonin uptake
Dextroamphetamine	better	better	worse	worse	worse	Inhibits NE and DA uptake
Levoamphetamine	better (animals)	No Δ	?	No Δ	?	Inhibits DA uptake
Lithium	?worse	?	better	?	?better	? ↓ NE release; ↑ NE uptake
Reserpine	worse	worse	better	better	better	Releases all stored biogenic amines
α Methyl paratyrosine	worse	?	better	?better	better	Prevents DA and NE synthesis
Physostigmine	worse	?	better	?	better	Antiacetylcholinesterase (effect on amines not studied yet)

It has thus far been difficult to isolate the behavioral effects of one amine from those of others because excesses of one cause alterations in the biological activity of the others. The effects of these drugs and their major mechanisms of action are summarized in Tables 5-1 and 5-2.

Table 5-2
Drugs, Movement, Mood, and Psychosis

	Parkinson's	Chorea	Depression	Psychosis
Better				
Primary	Belladonna L-dopa Amantadine	Reserpine Phenothiazines Major tranquilizers	MAOI Tricyclics	Reserpine Phenothiazines Major tranquilizers
Secondary	Amphetamine MAOI Tricyclics		Amphetamines ?L-dopa ?Belladonna	
Worse	Reserpine Phenothiazines Major Tranquilizers	L-dopa Amphetamines Belladonna Tricyclics	Reserpine Phenothiazines Major tranquilizers Amphetamine withdrawal	Amphetamines Belladonna Amantadine L-dopa MAOI Tricyclics

REFERENCES

Abraham, H. C., U. B. Kanter, I. Rosen, and J. L. Standen.   A controlled clinical trial of imipramine (Tofranil) with outpatients. Brit. J. Psychiat. 109: 286, 1963.

Angst, J., P. We's, P. C. Baastrup, and M. Schou.   Lithium prophylaxis in recurrent affective disorders. Brit. J. Psychiat. 116: 604-14, 1970.

Aquilonius, S. M. and R. Sjöström. Cholinergic and dopaminergic mechanisms in Huntington's chorea. Life Sciences 10: 405, 1971.

Baastrup, P. C. and M. Schou. Lithium as a prophylactic agent against recurrent depressions and manic depressive psychosis. Arch. Gen. Psychiat. 16: 162-72, 1967.

——, J. C. Poulsen, M. Schou, K. Thomsen, and A. Amdisen. Prophylactic lithium: double-blind discontinuation in manic depressive and recurrent depressive disorders. Lancet, New York, 1970, pp. 326-30.

Barbeau, A. Discussion. Association for Research in Nervous and Mental Disease. Neurotransmitters. December 1970.

Bartels, E. C. and O. Kuskacioglu. Narcolepsy: a possible cause of automobile accidents. Lahey Clin. Found. Bull. 14: 21, 1965.

Beck, A. T., C. H. Ward, M. Mandelson, J. Mock, and J. K. Erbaugh. Arch. Gen. Psychiat. 4: 561-70, 1961.

Bernheimer, H. and O. Hornykiewicz. Brain amines in Huntington's chorea. In: A. Barbeau, T. N. Chase, and G. W. Paulson, eds., Advances in Neurology Vol. 1, p. 525, 1973.

Biegel, A. and D. L. Murphy. Unipolar and bipolar affective illnesses. Arch. Gen. Psychiat. 24: 215-20, 1971.

Birkmayer, W. Der α methyl p tyrosine effekt bei extrapyramidalen erkrankungen. Wien. Klin. Wochensch. 81: 10, 1969.

Blumenthal, M. P. Heterogeneity and research on depressive disorders. Arch. Gen. Psychiat. 24: 524-31, 1971.

Buchsbaum, M., F. Goodwin, D. Murphy, and G. Borge. AER in affective disorders. Am. J. Psychiat. 128: 19-25, 1971.

Bunney, W. E., Jr., H. K. H. Brodie, D. L. Murphy, and F. K. Goodwin. Studies of alpha methyl paratyrosine, L-dopa and L tryptophan in depression and mania. Am. J. Psychiat. 127: 7, 1971.

Carlsson, A., H. Corrodi, K. Fuxe, T. Hökfelt. Effect of antidepressant drugs on the depletion of intraneuronal brain 5-hydroxytryptamine stores caused by 4 methyl α ethyl meta tyramine. Europ. J. Pharmacol. 5: 357, 1969.

Carman, J. B. Anatomic basis of surgical treatment of Parkinson's disease. New Eng. J. Med. 279: 919, 1968.

Carrea, R. M. E. and F. A. Mettler. Functions of the primate brachium conjunctivum and related structures. J. Comp. Neurol. 102: 151, 1955.

Chase, T. N. Biochemical and pharmacologic studies of monoamines in Huntington's chorea. Advances in Neurology Vol. 1. Raven Press, New York, 1973, p. 533.

Coppen, A.   The biochemistry of affective disorders. Brit. J. Psychiat. 113: 1237-64, 1967.

Cooper, I. S.   Involuntary Movement Disorders. Harper & Row, New York, 1968.

Cooper, J. R., F. E. Bloom, and R. H. Roth.   The Biochemical Basis of Neuropharmacology. Oxford University Press, New York, 1970.

Cotzias, G. C., P. S. Papavasiliou, and R. Gellene.   Modification of Parkinsonism—chronic treatment with L-dopa. New Eng. J. Med. 280: 337, 1969.

Coyle, J. T. and S. H. Snyder.   Antiparkinsonian drugs: Inhibition of dopamine uptake in the corpus striatum as a possible mechanism of action. Science 166: 899, 1969.

Curzon, G.   Relationships between stress and brain 5-hydroxytryptamine and their possible significance in affective disorders. In: B. Y. Ho and W. M. McIsaac, eds., Brain Chemistry and Mental Disease. Plenum, New York, 1971, pp. 163-176.

Davies, R., G. J. Tucker, M. Harrow, and T. Detre.   Confusional episodes and antidepressant medication. Amer. J. Psychiat. 128: 95-99, 1971.

Davis, J. M., D. S. Janowsky, and M. K. El-Yousef.   The use of lithium in clinical psychiatry. Psychiat. Annals 3: 78-99, 1973.

―――― and W. E. Fann,   Lithium. Ann. Rev. Pharmacol. 11: 285, 1971.

Dement, W., A. Rechtschaffen, and G. Gulevich.   The nature of the narcoleptic sleep attack. Neurology 16: 18, 1966.

Detre, T., J. Himmelhoch, M. Swartzburg, C. M. Anderson, R. Byck, and D. J. Kupfer. Hypersomnia and manic depressive disease. Am. J. Psychiat. 128: 1303, 1972.

――――, and H. Jarecki.   Modern Psychiatric Treatment. J. P. Lippincott Co., Philadelphia, 1971.

Donnelly, E. F. and T. N. Chase.   Intellectual and memory function in parkinsonian and non-parkinsonian patients treated with L-dopa. Dis. Nerv. System. 34: 119-23, 1973.

English, O. S. and S. M. Finch.   Introduction to Psychiatry. W. W. Norton and Co., New York, 1954.

Farnebo, L. O., K. Fuxe, M. Goldstein, B. Hamberger, and U. Ungerstedt.   Dopamine and noradrenaline releasing action of amantadine in the central and peripheral nervous system: a possible mode of action in Parkinson's disease. Europ. J. Pharmacol. 16: 27, 1971.

Freeman, J. M., A. M. Aron, J. E. Collard, and M. C. MacKay.   The emotional correlates of Syndenham's chorea. Pediatrics 35: 42, 1965.

Friedhoff, A. J. and E. Van Winkle. Characteristics of amine found in urine of schizophrenic patients. J. Nerv. and Ment. Dis. 135: 550, 1962.

Garron, D. C., H. L. Klawans, and F. Narin. Intellectual functioning of persons with idiopathic parkinsonism. J. Nerv. and Ment. Dis. 154: 445-52, 1972.

Goldberg, S. C., G. C. Klerman, and J. O. Cole. Changes in schizophrenic psychopathology and ward behavior as a function of phenothiazine treatment. Brit. J. Psychiat. 111: 120, 1965.

Goodman, L. S. and A. Gilman. The Pharmacological Basis of Therapeutics. 4th Edition. Macmillan Co., London, 1970.

Greenblatt, M., G. H. Grosser, and H. Wechsler. Differential response of hospitalized depressed patients to somatic therapy. Am. J. Psychiat. 120: 935, 1964.

Hamilton, M. Standardized assessment and recording of depressive symptoms. Psychiat. Neurol. Neuroclin. 72: 201, 1969.

Hartmann, E. Longitudinal studies of sleep and dream patterns in manic-depressive patients. Arch. Gen. Psychiat. 19: 311, 1968.

Hawkins, D. R. and J. Mendels. Sleep disturbance in depressive syndromes. Am. J. Psychiat. 123: 682-90, 1966.

Heathfield, K. W. G. Huntington's chorea: investigation into the prevalence of this disease in the area covered by the North East Metropolitan Regional Hospital Board. Brain 90: 203, 1967.

Hill, D. Depression: disease, reaction or posture. Am. J. Psychiat. 125: 445-57, 1968.

Himwich, H. E. and H. S. Alpers. Psychopharmacology. Ann. Rev. Pharmacol. 10: 313, 1970.

Hishikawa, Y., H. Ida, K. Nakai, and Z. Kaneko. Treatment of narcolepsy with imipramine (Tofranil) and desmethylimipramine (Pertofran). J. Neurol. Sci. 3: 453, 1966.

Hornykiewicz, O. Dopamine (3 hydroxytyramine) and brain function. Pharmac. Rev. 18: 925, 1966.

———. Dopamine and extrapyramidal motor function and dysfunction. Presented at ARNMD meeting, New York, 1970.

Janowsky, D. S., M. K. El-Yousef, J. M. Davis, and J. Sekerke. Parasympathetic suppression of manic symptoms by physostigmine. Arch. Gen. Psychiat. 28: 542-47, 1973.

———, ———, ———, ———, D. R. Morris, and B. Decker. Effects of amantadine on tardive dyskinesia and pseudo-Parkinsonism. New Eng. J. Med. 286: 784, 1972.

Jouvet, M. Neurophysiology of the States of Sleep. In: G. C. Quarton, T. Melnechuk, and F. O. Schmitt, eds., The Neurosciences: A Study Program. Rockefeller University Press, New York, 1967, p. 529.

Kallman, F. J. The genetics of psychoses: an analysis of 1232 twin index families. Internat. Cong. Psychiat. Rapports. 6: 1, 1950.

Kendell, R. E. The Classification of Depressive Illness. Oxford University Press, London, 1968.

Kety, S. S. Current biochemical approaches to schizophrenia. New Eng. J. Med. 276: 325, 1967.

Kiloh, L. C. and R. F. Garside. The independence of neurotic depression and endogenous depression. Brit. J. Psychiat. 109: 451, 1963.

Klawans, H. L. Jr. A pharmacologic analysis of Huntington's chorea. European Neurology 4: 148, 1970.

———, G. G. Paulsson, S. P. Ringel, and A. Barbeau. Use of L-dopa in the detection of presymptomatic Huntington's chorea. New Eng. J. Med. 286: 1332, 1972.

——— and R. Rubovits. Central cholinergic-anticholinergic antagonism in Huntington's chorea. Neurology 22: 107, 1972.

Klein, D. F. and J. M. Davis. Diagnosis and Drug Treatment of Psychiatric Disorders. Williams & Wilkins Co., Baltimore, 1969.

Kuhn, R. The treatment of depressive states with G22 355 (imipramine hydrochloride). Am. J. Psychiat. 115: 459, 1958.

Mindham, R. H. S. Psychiatric symptoms in Parkinsonism. J. Neurol. Neurosurg. Psychiat. 33: 188-91, 1970.

Murphy, D. L., H. K. Brodie, and F. K. Goodwin. Regular induction of hypomania by L-dopa in "bipolar" manic-depressive patients. Nature 229: 135-36, 1971.

Noyes, A. P. and L. C. Kolb. Modern Clinical Psychiatry. 6th Ed. W. B. Saunders Co., Philadelphia, 1963.

Parkes, C. M. The first year of bereavement. Psychiat. 33: 444-67, 1970.

Pollitt, J. D. Suggestions for a physiologic classification of depression. Brit. J. Psychiat. 111: 489-95, 1965.

Riklan, M. and E. Levita. Subcortical Correlates of Human Behavior. Williams & Wilkins Co., Baltimore, 1969.

Robins, E. and S. Guze. Classification of affective disorders. In: Recent Advances in the Psychobiology of the Depressive Illnesses. DHEW Publication No. 70-9053, 1972, pp. 283-93. U.S. Government Printing Office, Washington, D.C.

Sachar, E. J. Corticosteroids in depressive illness. Arch. Gen. Psychiat. 17: 544-67, 1967.

Schildkraut, J. J. Neurochemical studies of the affective disorders. Am. J. Psychiat. 127: 358-60, 1970.

————. Norepinephrine metabolites as biochemical criteria for classifying depressive disorders and predicting responses to treatment. Am. J. Psychiat. 130: 695-99, 1973.

Schwab, R. S., H. D. Fabing, and J. S. Pritchard. Psychiatric symptoms and syndromes in Parkinson's disease. Am. J. Psychiat. 107: 901-7, 1951.

Slater, E. and V. Cowie. The Genetics of Mental Disorders. Oxford University Press, London, 1971.

Small, J. C., I. F. Small, and D. F. Moore. Experimental withdrawal of lithium in recovered manic-depressive patients. Am. J. Psychiat. 127: 131-34, 1971.

Snyder, S. H. Psychoactive drugs and central neurotransmitters. Presented at Assoc. for Res. in Nerv. and Ment. Dis., New York City, 1970.

Sours, J. A. Narcolepsy and other disturbances in the sleep waking rhythm: a study of 115 cases with review of the literature. J. Nerv. Ment. Dis. 147: 525, 1963.

Sulser, F. and E. Sanders-Bush. Effect of drugs on amines in the CNS. Ann. Rev. Pharmacol. 11: 209, 1971.

Taylor, K. M. and S. H. Snyder. Amphetamine: differentiation by d and l isomers of behavior involving brain norepinephrine or dopamine. Science 168: 1487, 1970.

———— and ————. Differential effects of d and l amphetamine on behavior and on catecholamine disposition in dopamine and norepinephrine-containing neurons of rat brain. Brain Res. 28: 295, 1971.

Van Woert, M. H., L. M. Ambani, and M. B. Bowers Jr. Levodopa and cholinergic hypersensitivity in Parkinson's disease. Neurology 22: 86, 1972.

Weintraub, M. I. and M. H. Van Woert. Reversal of cholinergic hypersensitivity in Parkinson's disease by levodopa. New Eng. J. Med. 284: 412, 1971.

Whatmore, G. B. and R. M. Ellis. Further neurophysiologic aspects of depressed states. Arch. Gen. Psychiat. 6: 243-53, 1962.

Whittier, J., G. Haydu, and J. Crawford. Effect of imipramine (Tofranil) on depression and hyperkinesia in Huntington's disease. Am. J. Psychiat. 118: 79, 1961.

Whybrow, P. C. and J. Mendels. Towards a biology of depression: some suggestions from neurophysiology. Am. J. Psychiat. 125: 1491-1500, 1969.

Winokur, G., R. Cadoret, J. Dorzab, and M. Baker.   Depressive disease: a genetic study. Arch. Gen. Psychiat. 24: 135-44, 1971.

Wittenborn, J. R., M. Plante, F. Burgess, and H. Maurer.   A comparison of imipramine, electroconvulsive therapy and placebo in the treatment of depressions. J. Nerv. Ment. Dis. 135: 131, 1962.

Wyatt, R. J., D. H. Fram, R. Buchbinder, and F. Snyder.   Treatment of intractable narcolepsy with a monamine oxidase inhibitor. New Eng. J. Med. 285: 987, 1971.

Yahr, M. D. and R. C. Duvoisin.   Drug therapy of Parkinsonism. New Eng. J. Med. 287: 20, 1972.

Yaryura-Tobias, J. A., B. Diamond, and S. Merlis.   The action of L-dopa on schizophrenic patients (A preliminary report) Curr. Ther. Res. 12: 528, 1970.

Zarcone, V.   Narcolepsy. New Eng. J. Med. 288: 1156, 1973.

Zung, W. K. K.   A self rating depression scale. Arch. Gen. Psychiat. 12: 63, 1965.

Chapter 6

MANIFESTATIONS OF ANXIETY

While the entities dealt with in this section—hysteria, hyperventilation, headache, and chronic hypochondriasis—seem disparate, they are quite similar in several ways. All these conditions are common and often coexist or appear over the years in affected individuals. They are clear examples of how an alteration in mental function can lead to physiologic change. While classified as neurotic disorders, they may be seen in patients with serious neurological and other medical diseases, in schizophrenics, in depressed persons, and in individuals whose personalities are dominated by them in a chronic, unremitting, nonprogressive fashion throughout life. They form a syndrome, in other words, the prognosis of which depends upon the basic conditions with which they are associated.

HYPERVENTILATION SYNDROME

Of all psychophysiological reactions probably the most common one dealt with by physicians is the hyperventilation syndrome (HVS). Because its manifestations in different body systems can mimic other conditions, this syndrome is frequently unrecognized and patients are often shunted from doctor to doctor undergoing numerous diagnostic tests which are unnecessary and upsetting. Often the result of anxiety, hyperventilation produces changes in body functions which themselves become the focus of anxiety. Fear and confusion are compounded when a doctor tells his patient that his symptoms are factitious, "all in his nerves." The patient knows his symptoms are not imagined and supposes he has a life-threatening illness. The symptoms of hyperventilation syndrome include faintness, visual disturbances, inability to concentrate, nausea, vertiginous instability, headache, fullness in the head and chest and epigastrium, breathlessness, palpitations, hot flushing, cold sweating, paresthesias, and occasionally vomiting. This panoply of symptoms results from physiological alterations that can be caused simply by overbreathing.

A study of the hyperventilation syndrome in neurologic practice was undertaken by reviewing the charts of the 550 patients seen by one of us (JHP) over a five year period at the Yale New Haven Hospital in the private out-patient neurology clinic.* All referred patients were suspected of having a neurological condition. Age, sex, past medical history, present symptoms, and past history of psychosomatic illnesses were noted. The diagnosis of HVS was made on the basis of the patient's response to overbreathing. Each patient who complained of any of the symptoms associated with HVS was asked to overbreathe by mouth for up to three minutes or until he became dizzy. If the symptoms of which he complained were thus reproduced in their entirety and if no other explanation for the symptoms could be adduced from physical examination, medical history or laboratory tests, the diagnosis was considered established.

Thirty patients met these criteria. They ranged in age from fifteen to sixty years. In order to ascertain whether HVS was more prevalent at certain ages and among women, a control group of 58 patients was randomly selected from the remaining 520 for detailed review, and these were fairly evenly distributed between the ages of several months to 75. Eighty-six per cent of the study group but only 24 per cent of the control group were between the ages of

---

* The data quoted were derived from the student thesis of Bruce B. Haak at the Yale University School of Medicine.

fifteen and thirty (p < .01). Eighty-seven per cent of the study group but only 49 per cent of the control group were women (p < .05) (Table 6-1). Twenty-nine per cent of all women re-

Table 6-1
Patients with Hyperventilation Syndrome and Neurologic Controls* by Age and Sex

Age	0-15	15-30	30-45	45-60	60-75	Total
HVS (M)	0	2	1	1	0	4
(F)	0	16	5	5	0	26
						30
Control*						
(M)	7	8	3	5	7	30
(F)	5	6	6	6	5	28
						58

* Controls were drawn at random from the same private neurologic outpatient clinic population of 550 from which the 30 patients with HVS had been drawn.

Table 6-2
Incidence of Psychosomatic Illness* in Patients with Hyperventilation Syndrome and Neurologic Controls by Age and Sex

Age	0-15	15-30	30-45	45-60	60-75	Total
HVS (M)	0	1/2	1/1	1/1	0/0	3/4
(F)	0	13/16	5/5	2/5	0/0	20/26
Control						
(M)	1/7	1/8	1/3	0/5	1/7	4/30
(F)	0/5	2/6	3/6	5/6	1/5	11/28

* Psychosomatic illness was taken to mean a previous history of medical symptoms the investigation of which produced negative results or conversion reactions, and/or multiple visits to physicians for minor problems (hypochondriasis).

ferred for neurological consultation between ages fifteen and thirty had HVS as the sole cause of their chief complaint. This was true of less than 5 per cent of the men in the same age group.

A history of psychosomatic illness in the past was more common in the study group. This term encompasses complicated medical symptoms with negative evaluations, conversion reactions, psychophysiologic reactions and multiple visits to physicians for minor conditions (hypochondriasis). Seventy-seven per cent of the patients with HVS had a history of psychosomatic illness in the past as compared with 28 per cent in the control group ($p < .05$). Psychosomatic illness was twice as prevalent among women with HVS aged 15-45 as among control women of the same age ($p < .05$).

The chief complaints of the study group were usually multiple and included lightheadedness (80%), paresthesias (50%), headache (37%), weakness (27%), breathlessness (23%), inability to swallow (23%), inability to concentrate (23%), palpitations (20%), chest pains (17%), abdominal pains (10%), loss of consciousness (6%), tetany (3%).

The mechanism by which hyperventilation causes such symptoms is the lowering of pCO_2. Five deep breaths produced by yawning or sighing are enough to alter pCO_2 significantly and produce symptoms (Plum and Posner, 1972). The lowered pCO_2 reduces cerebral blood flow for there is a direct relation between pCO_2 and the caliber of cerebral blood vessels. In 240 seconds of overbreathing cerebral blood flow can be reduced by 40 per cent. Thus, hyperventilation leads to cerebral hypoxia and this is the cause of the EEG slowing so often seen with overbreathing (Gotoh et al., 1965). Prolonged hyperventilation can produce respiratory alkalosis, which in turn can induce tetany.

Hyperventilation is a routine part of electroencephalographic testing and may induce an epileptiform abnormality. Of course, it can also induce actual seizures. Hyperventilation in response to anxiety may in fact be a major mechanism by which emotional tension induces seizures in susceptible individuals (Mattson et al.,

1970). The cerebral hypoxia caused by hyperventilation when compounded by a mild degree of orthostatic hypotension and/or the Valsalva maneuver may reduce cerebral blood flow to the degree that the patient faints or has a convulsion. (Many young boys have learned to induce syncope by overbreathing and then performing the Valsalva maneuver for the amusement of their friends.)

Hyperventilation can also cause nonspecific ST- and T-wave changes in the electrocardiogram (Christensen, 1946) and many HVS patients showing such EKG changes have been admitted to coronary care units. Hyperventilation is often associated with air swallowing and this, in turn, can lead to epigastric distress.

Hyperventilation is a very common response to anxiety. One might almost call it a universal human reaction to anxiety for it is part of the autonomic response to threatening situations. That it becomes a symptom which leads people to seek medical attention primarily when they are predisposed to conversion reaction, hypochondriasis, or psychosomatic illnesses is suggested by our finding a history of such previous problems in more than ¾ of HVS patients. Young women aged fifteen to thirty seem to be particularly susceptible. Preadolescents and patients at retirement age appear to be less so.

Seven of the 30 patients with HVS had organic diseases as well, including regional ileitis, adrenal insufficiency, and peptic ulcer. Of these seven, five were more than thirty years of age. For this reason it would seem prudent, especially in patients over thirty years of age, to consider the possibility of associated medical illnesses even in the face of HVS.

HEADACHE

Determining the cause of headache is one of the most important diagnoses a physician has to make. Headache can be a symptom of anxiety or depression or it can be the first symptom of a brain tumor. It is not our purpose to provide here a comprehensive discussion of headache. For this the reader is referred to the excellent books by Wolff and Dalessio (1972) and Friedman and Merritt (1959). We will merely put forward the criteria from the patient's history that are helpful in distinguishing headaches of psychogenic origin from those of neurologic origin.

Headaches which are dull, generalized, and constant for many days in a row almost invariably have no neurological cause. Patients with such headaches often describe "a pressure feeling" which is what they mean by headaches. These patients almost always have an impressive past history of psychosomatic illness and are depressed. The unremitting character of the headaches and the patient's complaints of their severity usually contrast with the fact that he is nonetheless able to work. Analgesics, tranquilizers, and sedatives are usually ineffective but antidepressants often help. In general, headaches of sudden onset, headaches that awaken a patient from sleep, or unilateral headaches are not caused by purely emotional factors.

Tension headaches are caused by muscle tension. When the muscles in the posterior neck and temples are under the stress of continuous contraction, they begin to produce the symptom of aching just as muscles anywhere in the body do when they have been overworked. The pain reflection is then generalized over the head. Such headaches are dull and steady though occasionally a sustained muscle contraction headache is followed by a typical vascular (throbbing) headache and the two types of headache coexist in an attack. Tension-type headaches can usually be attributed to emotional tension but sometimes cervical pathology such as osteoarthritis or cervical disc disease is the cause by secondarily producing the cervical muscle contractions. Tension headaches characteristically occur in the morning on awakening or in the late afternoon. These headaches are worse during the working week and tend to be relieved on weekends and vacations. They are generally relieved by aspirin and sedatives. Tension headaches are often mistakenly attributed to essential hypertension or chronic sinusitis. With few exceptions, by the time a patient comes to a doctor for treatment of tension headaches, he will have had them for months or years. Surprisingly this holds true for children too. Some patients who initially deny the longstanding nature of their headaches when pressed will admit that they have had similar headaches in the past, though perhaps not as severe or as frequent. This point is important in distinguishing ordinary tension headaches from those caused by brain tumors.

Headaches are caused by brain tumors in two ways, by increased intracranial pressure and by traction of the mass on pain-sensitive structures within the skull. No single headache is characteristic of a brain tumor. Headaches caused by increased intracranial pressure are, if anything, remarkable for being nonspecific. They are mild, dull, aching, and very often bifrontal or bioccipital. They may be present in the morning on awakening, last a few hours, and get better as the day goes on. They may not occur every day. Thus, they may be quite similar to tension headaches. Headaches produced by increased intracranial pressure, however, are characteristically of recent onset, usually starting within a few weeks before the patient presents himself to the physician. We have found this to be the most important feature in distinguishing tension headaches from those caused by increased intracranial pressure.

When brain tumors cause headaches by traction on pain-sensitive structures, headaches are often lateralized or localized to one spot. Intraventricular tumors can cause headaches which may be exacerbated or relieved by changes in position. Thus, any time a patient complains of a headache which is brought on by putting his head in one position and relieved by changing the position, a mechanical factor must be considered and the possibility of a tumor investigated thoroughly.

Headaches which follow the performance of a lumbar puncture are mechanical in origin too and result from traction on pain-sensitive structures at the base of the brain after loss of spinal fluid which normally cushions these structures from the skull beneath.

Reclining in a supine position promptly relieves such headaches. Contrary to common belief, emotional factors do not play an important role in producing these headaches.

Prostrating headaches that are throbbing and severe, last several hours, and are associated with photophobia, scintillations, nausea, and vomiting are usually migrainous. This is so whether or not they are unilateral or are preceded by typical ischemic symptoms such as flashing lights, scintillating scotomata, or sensory or motor symptoms. Patients with such prostrating headaches usually have a positive family history of migraine, which suggests a hereditary factor. Migraine headaches occur primarily in the young, often begin in the first decade, and hardly ever develop after the age of thirty years. They may tend to occur more frequently on weekends and vacations and are unaffected by ordinary analgesics. Contrary to popular belief, emotional factors usually play a minor role in the etiology of migraine headaches and psychotherapy usually does not relieve them. Ergot-containing preparations are usually effective in stopping such headaches if they are taken in the early stages of the attack, especially during the prodrome.

Another form of headache that is common but perhaps little known to psychiatrists often follows minor or major head trauma. This occurs in the "post-traumatic" syndrome, a form of traumatic encephalopathy, which also involves giddiness, irritability, sensitivity to noise, and minor memory and concentration difficulties. Lishman (1968) noted that the occurrence of the symptoms was unrelated to either the extent or location of brain damage. Jacobsen (1969) however noted that these symptoms were more likely to occur if the patient was rendered unconscious at the time of impact. He observed that the headaches usually stopped within two months of the injury and that most patients were free of all symptoms within four years. This syndrome is not usually associated with radiographic or electroencephalographic changes and many have questioned its organic basis, suggesting that the symptoms resolve, "when the lawsuit arising from the injury is settled (two months to four years usually)." The distinctiveness of the syndrome argues against this "psychosomatic" view of its etiology, in our opinion, as does the fact that it may occur in individuals with no history of psychosomatic disease or pending lawsuits.

HYSTERIA

Hysteria is a much abused word. It can be used to refer to a personality type or to a psychosomatic reaction (conversion) or as a pejorative term indicating a generalized, disorganized response to stress, e.g., hysterical. The hysterical personality has been described as vain, egocentric, labile, excitable, dramatic, attention-seeking, overly conscious of sex, provocative but frigid, dependent, and demanding. Although this label is applied to both men and women it is most often attached to attractive, overly made-up, seductive and exhibitionistic women. It is a fairly common personality type. In those who manifest (hysterical) conversion symptoms, however, the hysterical personality type is relatively uncommon and is seen in roughly one-fifth of patients with conversion symptoms (Ljungberg, 1957). Conversion symptoms are probably more prevalent in people with hysterical personalities than in the general population, but this is by no means an obligatory association (Chodoff, 1958; Zeigler et al., 1960; Zeigler and Imboden, 1962).

Our discussion of hysteria will be limited to those conversion reactions that can be confused with neurologic illnesses. By conversion reactions we mean loss or impairment of normal functions which does not result from physiological abnormalities. We have found that two criteria are extremely important in making a positive diagnosis of conversion reaction. Unless both are present the diagnosis should be held in doubt. These criteria are: (1) That there must be no organic lesion which can explain the patient's symptoms and (2) That there must be (even in children) a past history of conversion reactions, hypochondriasis, or psychophysiologic reactions. The latter term refers to physiologically based dysfunctions which are caused largely by emotional factors, e.g., neuro-dermatitis, peptic ulcer, spastic colon, hyperventilation syndrome. The importance of these criteria was most clearly delineated by Perley and Guze (1962), who were among the first to stipulate and validate them. When the two criteria are used, hysteria appears to be a distinct syndrome.

Perley and Guze studied a group of 39 patients who met these criteria for six to eight years. Ninety per cent of their patients did not develop any other illness which might have explained the symptoms. The patients' tendency to develop further psychosomatic conditions continued over the years. This study called attention to the importance of a complete and detailed history in dealing with patients suspected of conversion reactions.

Slater and Glithero (1965) made a retrospective study of 85 patients diagnosed as hysterical by various clinicians (presumably on the basis of various criteria) after ten years had passed. Of the 85 patients with a chart diagnosis of hysteria, they found on follow-up that 22 had later been given a diagnosis of organic disease which could have explained their initial symptoms. At the time they were diagnosed as hysterical 19 of the patients had medical illnesses which could have explained their symptoms. Four patients had committed suicide, and eight had died of their medical conditions. Well over half the total population of "hysterics" had medical problems that were mistaken as psychogenic or that had precipitated emotional reactions. This study indicates the need for cautious and precise diagnosis, which the following case confirms:

A 55 year old factory worker had been involved in an industrial accident which injured his back. He had worked for the same company for 15 years and had only rare absences for illness. There was no history of psychiatric or psychosomatic illness. There was a compensation suit pending. The patient was referred to the Department of Orthopedics for evaluation of his back. X-rays showed minor changes of the body of the 12th dorsal vertebra which could have been related to trauma, neoplasm, or infection and it was decided to perform a punch biopsy of that vertebra. One hour after the performance of the biopsy, the patient announced blandly and calmly that he would never walk again. Examination revealed total paraplegia, depressed tendon reflexes in the lower extremities, and normal touch, pinprick, vibration, and position sensation. His obvious indifference to his circumstances, the clear "secondary gain" and the inability of his physicians to explain how a lesion which destroyed all motor function below the first lumbar segments could fail to cause any sensory symptoms led to the diagnosis of "conversion reaction or malingering." Eight hours after the biopsy, he developed a sensory level of hypalgesia below L1. A myelogram was performed which demonstrated a complete block and shortly after the myelogram was done he went into shock and died. At autopsy it was found that he had a metastatic carcinoma of the lung which had invaded his 12th dorsal vertebral body. The punch biopsy had caused extensive hemorrhage that compressed his cord.

Of key importance in this case was the absence of any previous tendency toward hypochondriasis, psychosomatic, or conversion reaction. Because of the physicians' inexperience "la belle indifference," "secondary gain," and neurological findings which "could not be explained" led them to make the diagnosis of hysteria in error. The two classical hallmarks of hysteria, "la belle indifference" and "secondary gain," have been, in our experience, more often misleading than helpful in establishing the diagnosis.

Apparent indifference is often a sign of stoicism and stoical hospitalized patients are more often seriously ill than hysterical. Hysterical patients may be excited and anxious when they develop conversion symptoms, though it is true that many do manifest "la belle indifference."

The secondary gain, which refers to the reward of the patient who develops a conversion reaction, is often difficult to identify. Sometimes it is no more than staying in the hospital and avoiding contact with the family; sometimes it may be a more subtle, even a fantasized gain. On the other hand, patients who have been injured in automobile or industrial accidents often have lawsuits or compensation claims pending which are quite justified but could be incorrectly thought to represent "secondary gain" by their physicians.

It has been our experience that most medical doctors consider a patient hysterical only when they cannot imagine an organic lesion that could explain his symptoms. Mistakes are made because the physician's diagnostic acumen is naturally a function of his previous experience and knowledge. No one can know everything, and peculiar facets of difficult cases of organic disease can appear which even the most experienced clinician has not encountered before. It may be worthwhile to consider some of the classic conversion symptoms which masquerade as neurologic conditions in relation to the inadequacy of the criterion that no organic lesion can be imagined to explain the symptoms as the sole basis for a diagnosis of hysteria.

Inability to swallow or feeling a lump in the throat is typical of "globus hystericus." Normal results on direct examination of the nasal and oral pharynx and on barium swallow studies are sufficient to rule out most lesions which could give similar symptoms. On the other hand, both myasthenia gravis and polymyositis may begin with intermittent weakness of the swallowing mechanism. At the time of examination the patient may be able to swallow normally and may appear to be well. Similarly, pseudobulbar palsy, which interferes with swallowing may wax and wane in severity. When unassociated with other signs of neurologic disease, such symptoms have been mistakenly considered hysterical.

Typical visual conversion symptoms include monocular diplopia and tunnel vision. Though monocular diplopia is in most cases caused by hysteria, ocular pathology such as dislocated lenses and parietal lobe lesions can give rise to it (Kestenbaum, 1961). Tunnel vision is also typically caused by hysteria, but something similar may develop in both syphilis and glaucoma.

Hysterical hemisensory loss usually involves half the entire body, from head to feet and from the extremities to the midline. A pinprick is not felt on one side of the linea alba but will be felt normally on the other side. The sensory splitting at the exact midline is considered by many to be a hard and fast sign of hysteria since organic hemisensory deficits typically appear 1 or 2 centimeters to the right or left of midline. It is also said that the diagnosis of hysteria can be confirmed by testing vibratory sensation on the skull. A tuning fork placed upon the skull to one side of midline should be felt by neurological patients no matter which side the hemisensory loss is on because the oscillations of the tuning fork are transmitted throughout the entire skull. If the patient does not feel vibrations, he may be considered hysterical.

Unfortunately, these sensory signs of hysteria are rather unreliable because some patients with neurologic diseases report what they think their examiner wishes them to report and claim that a change in sensation occurs at the midline when in fact this is not so. In addition, it is conceivable that a minority of patients have a physiologically variant pattern of sensory functioning in which the anesthesia caused by brain lesion does in fact change at the midline. Also patients who report absent vibratory sensation on the anesthetic side of their skulls may in fact feel vibrations less on that side but report to the examiner that they feel nothing to be "consistent."

Hysterical hemiplegia may be diagnosed in the following way: placing his hands underneath the patient's paralyzed heel while the patient is supine, the examiner asks the patient to raise his normal leg. The examiner can thereby determine whether or not the patient is able to move his paralyzed leg because the normal response while raising one leg is to push down with the other. If the patient pushes down with his "paralyzed" leg, the factitious nature of his paralysis should be clear. By reversing the process and asking the patient to raise the paralyzed leg, the examiner can determine whether or not the patient is actually trying to lift it. If the patient does not push down with the good leg, the examiner can conclude that he is not trying to raise the paralyzed leg. This test is only useful in complete hemiplegia, however, and will not help in discerning hysterical hemiparesis (which is more common than hysterical hemiplegia) from true hemiparesis. The presence of unilateral changes in deep tendon reflexes, spasticity, and Babinskis provides objective evidence indicating neurological disease. The absence of these alterations, however, cannot establish the diagnosis of hysteria.

Hysterical hemiparesis is characteristically associated with "give-way" weakness. By this phrase is meant discontinuous resistance during direct muscle testing. Give-way weakness is absolutely diagnostic of factitious weakness but occasionally a patient will exaggerate mild, real weakness in order to convince the examiner that he is, in fact, weak. In such cases, the patient may feel that the examiner is going to miss the diagnosis and so he "helps out" by exaggerating. Reflex abnormalities, when present, can rule out hysteria but the absence of such abnormalities will not establish the diagnosis.

Astasia-abasia or hysterical gait, can sometimes be extremely difficult to tell from movement disorders. Physicians routinely place emphasis on the following indications that a disordered gait is hysterical. The patient walks well when unaware that he is being observed, never falls, and does not injure himself. Since almost all movement disorders are worsened by anxiety, it is not wise to accept without reservation reports by nurses and other staff to the effect that the patient is able to walk nearly normally when unaware that he is being observed. If the patient is made nervous by an examiner or a large group of physicians on rounds and his movement disorder worsens, this is only natural. Sometimes patients with hysterical gait problems do, in fact, fall and may accidentally hurt themselves so that a history of falls with occasional scrapes and bruises does not necessarily rule out hysteria.

In our experience, most movement disorders, whether organic or hysterical, are likely to cause a certain amount of confusion amongst clinicians. It is not at all uncommon to find a minority of competent neurologists who will consider a given patient to be either organic or hysterical even in the face of an opposite majority view. Fortunately, there is a relatively safe and fairly objective test for hysteria in such cases: amytal infusion. Amytal is infused intravenously at a rate of 100 mg per 30 seconds until nystagmus develops. This usually requires 250 to 500 mgs. As soon as nystagmus develops, the infusion is stopped and the patient is asked to perform the motor task that he previously found difficult. If there is substantial improvement in his movement disorder, the diagnosis of hysteria is supported. If the gait deteriorates, the diagnosis of organicity is supported. This test is often extremely helpful but it can be misinterpreted. When anxiety is responsible for marked worsening of an organic movement disorder, amytal might occasionally improve the gait by relieving anxiety.

Hysterical amnesias, fugue states and pseudodementia can also cause diagnostic confusion. In previous chapters, particularly the one on epilepsy, we noted that transient fluctuations in consciousness can be associated with epileptic conditions and we suggested some guidelines for diagnosis (p. 21). Hysterical states may partially mimic epilepsy and can be confused with it. It is a rare psychiatrist or neurologist who has not been confronted with a patient who says he does not know who he is, or who he was at a particular time, or where he has come from. Such hysterical states are most often seen in times of stress, for instance, among soldiers during war or in individuals indicted for crimes. Characteristics that help to distinguish those with psychogenic amnesia or dissociative states from neurologic patients include the following: (1) In hysterical states the patients are able to carry out complex functions during the time of amnesia. (2) Memory loss and shift of identity to another person or personality are usually sudden. (3) The patient's behavior is fairly well integrated in that he usually has enough money to get where he is going and takes time to eat and drink. (4) Loss of memory usually affects a specific section of life or ability, i.e., arithmetic or recognition of certain relatives. (5) The transition to a normal state is abrupt. (6) There is no history or physical evidence of neurological disease. Yet even if all these characteristics indicate hysteria, unless the past history provides support for a psychosomatic tendency, the diagnosis should be held in doubt. Other conditions can cause "dissociative states."

Berrington studied 37 cases of fugue state and noted that depression was a frequent concomitant. Interestingly, he noted that a high proportion of the patients had a history of head injury and he speculated that this may have precipitated the fugue state. He also observed that the patients were usually completely unaware of their identity and past life and acted as if they were in a dream. During the episodes, they could travel and seemed able to answer complex questions adequately. They had either partial or complete amnesia for the episodes.

The syndrome of "transient global amnesia," described by Fisher and Adams (1958) and by Shuttleworth and Morris (1966) is marked by periods of confusion and disorientation to time and place that usually last a few hours. Patients in these two studies had no recollection of events and described themselves as feeling strange during the episodes of amnesia. In contrast to the above-mentioned syndromes of hysterical amnesia and fugue state, which usually affect individuals in the third or fourth decade, these patients were all middle-aged or elderly and had a history of hypertension or atherosclerosis. Although they did not lose their identity, they could not retain new information during these episodes. It was hypothesized that the episodes resulted from transient ischemia, specifically ischemia of the mamillary-hippocampal complex.

Perhaps it is fitting that we have concluded this book with a chapter that deals in part with hysteria. The syndrome was first studied by a neurologist, Charcot, and it provided a springboard for modern psychiatry through the work of one of his most illustrious pupils, Freud. It has been designated variously as a neurologic syndrome, a psychiatric syndrome, and a disease of society (Vieth, 1965). To a degree it crystallized the dilemma we have had in writing this book: we have had to constantly check ourselves from referring to psychiatric illnesses as "functional" thereby implying a separateness from "organic" illness that does not exist. It should be apparent that almost every abnormal emotional state can be produced by one or more neurologic syndromes. It is self-evident that all behavioral symptoms, whatever their etiology are mediated by the central nervous system, a common pathway for many different pathologic processes. Though most conversion syndromes exist in the absence of neurologic disease, one wonders why one patient and not another develops hysteria, in response to apparently similar life stresses. There is no clear answer to this problem yet. Genetic aspects have been incompletely explored and we have not been able to identify causative environmental influences. While our knowledge of hysterical conditions has increased considerably over the years (we no longer believe that the varied symptoms are related to a "wandering uterus" and we have been able to formulate criteria for the diagnosis), our skills are still exercised fundamentally at a descriptive level. This is true of many neurological and psychiatric conditions. While we look to basic medical research for the full understanding of these diseases, it behooves us meanwhile to polish our clinical skills and learn what we can from observation and description.

REFERENCES

Berrington, W. P., D. W. Liddell, and G. A. Foulds. A re-evaluation of the fugue. J. Ment. Sci. 102: 280, 1956.

Chodoff, P. and H. Lyons. Hysteria, the hysterical personality and "hysterical" conversion. Am. J. Psychiat. 114: 734, 1958.

Christensen, B. Studies on hyperventilation. II Electrocardiographic changes in normal man during voluntary hyperventilation. J. Clin. Invest. 24: 880, 1946.

Fisher, C. M. and R. D. Adams. Transient global amnesia. Acta Neurol. Scand. 40 (suppl 9): 7, 1964.

Friedman, A. P. and H. H. Merritt. Headache: Diagnosis and Treatment. F. A. Davis Co., Philadelphia, 1959.

Gotoh, F., J. S. Meyer, and Y. Takagi. Cerebral effects of hyperventilation in man. Arch. Neurol. 12: 410, 1965.

Jacobson, S. A. Mechanisms of the sequellae of minor craniocervical trauma. In: A. E. Walker, W. F. Caveness and M. Critchley, eds., The Late Effects of Head Injury. C. C. Thomas, Springfield, Ill., 1969, p. 35.

Kestenbaum, A.   Clinical Methods of Neuro-ophthalmologic Examination. 2nd ed. Grune and Stratton, New York, 1961.

Lishman, W. A.   Brain damage in relation to psychiatric disability after head injury. Brit. J. Psychiat. 114: 373, 1968.

Ljungberg, L.   Hysteria: a clinical, prognostic and genetic study. Acta Psychiat. Scand. Suppl. 112, 1957.

Mattson, R. H., G. R. Heninger, B. B. Gallagher, and G. H. Glaser. Psychophysiological precipitants of seizures in epileptics. Neurology 20: 406, 1970.

Perley, M. J. and S. B. Guze.   Hysteria—the stability and usefulness of clinical criteria. A quantitative study based on a follow-up of six to eight years in 39 patients. New Eng. J. Med. 266:421, 1962.

Plum, F. and J. B. Posner.   Diagnosis of Stupor and Coma. 2nd ed. Contemporary Neurology Series. F. A. Davis Co., Philadelphia, 1972.

Shuttleworth, E. C. and C. E. Morris.   The transient global amnesia syndrome. Arch. Neurol. 15: 515, 1966.

Slater, E. and E. Glithero.   A follow-up of patients diagnosed as suffering from "hysteria." J. Psychosom. Res. 9: 9, 1965.

Veith, I.   Hysteria. University of Chicago Press, Chicago, 1965.

Wolff, I. and D. J. Dalessio.   Headache and other head pain. 3rd ed. Oxford University Press, New York, 1972.

Ziegler, F. J., J. B. Imboden, and E. Meyer.   Contemporary conversion reactions: clinical study. Am. J. Psychiat. 116: 909, 1960.

———— and ————.   Contemporary conversion reactions II: Conceptual model. Arch. Gen. Psychiat. 66: 279, 1962.

INDEX